Medicine Flows

Homoeopathic Philosophy

by Mo Morrish

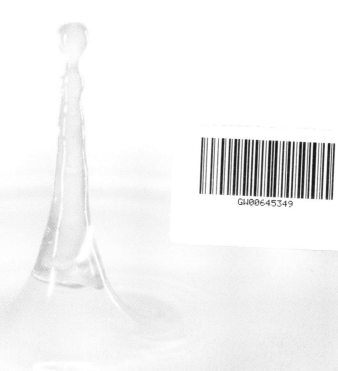

GW00645349

First Published in 2006 by Homoeopathy Centre Publications.

Web: www.homoeopathycentre.com

The right of Mo Morrish to be identified as the author of this work has been asserted by him in accordance with the Copyright, Designs and Patents Act 1988

ISBN 0 9552662 0 3

Editing by Delny Britton
Design and Typesetting by Sharon Kemmett, Isis Design
Printed and bound in the UK by Russell Press

Permission to quote has kindly been granted by Birdcage Books, B. Jain Publishers (P) Ltd. and Beaconsfield Publishers Ltd.

Whilst every effort has been made to ensure the accuracy of the information in this book the publisher and author accept no responsibility for any errors or omissions. Unsuccessful attempts have been made to contact a copyright owner: we would be pleased to hear from him/her.

Medicine Flows

Dedication

This is respectfully dedicated to the memory of Kenneth Metson who didn't so much teach as show me how simple and effective homoeopathic medicine can be.

Thanks maestro, I hope I can pass it on.

'Everything flows!'
Heraclitus

'The beauty of homoeopathy lies in its simplicity,
The power of homoeopathy lies in its depth,
The danger of homoeopathy lies in its shallow application.'
Paschero

'Take your well-disciplined strengths
and stretch them between two
opposing poles. Because inside human beings
is where God learns.'
Rilke

Contents

Part Four: THE HOMOEOPATH

Part Five: THE MEDICINES

Acknowledgements

A big 'thank you' to all the people I have worked with in clinic and in classroom, as patients and students: you have shown me how to practise and to teach.

Special thanks and respect go to Anthony Bickley for giving me the opportunity to teach and the freedom to find my way in that, and to the core team at the British School of Homoeopathy down the years, most especially Frank Meredith.

Warmest thanks to Jane Hurley for a homoeopathic friendship and for being a safe port in that storm.

Respect and appreciation go to Ian Watson for his insightful foreword and his own *Tao of Homeopathy*.

A huge 'thank you' goes to my homoeopathic community of peers for their time, encouragement and kind words. Sarah Bickley, Miranda Castro, Linda Gwillim, Anne Marshall, Claus Mikosch, John Morgan, Ray Nolan, Wenda Brewster O'Reilly, Saskia Ross, Ruth Sewell and Ian Webster.

In bringing the book together I offer special thanks to Delny Britton for a sharp eye and skillful editing; to Sharon Kemmett for dynamic design and endless patience; to Sally Tofton for publishing with assurance and style.

Lastly to my wife, Ali, for loving me, believing in me and making me laugh in almost all circumstances!

Thank you.

Foreword

Behind every discipline lies a set of core ideas and assumptions which the practitioner must assimilate and digest before he or she can fully embody their chosen vocation, and homoeopathy is no exception. There is a gulf of difference between *learning* homoeopathy and actually *becoming* a homoeopath, a process which requires the individual to perceive the world from a standpoint that is uniquely 'homoeopathic'.

The challenge every new practitioner faces is that of translating their homoeopathic understanding into a way of practising that is appropriate to their individual nature, faithful to homoeopathy's philosophical roots, and relevant to modern times. This is no easy task, and there are many who stumble between the cracks that seem to open up between theory and practice.

Mo brings a fresh perspective to Hahnemann's legacy that will enrich and deepen the understanding of student and practitioner alike. Weaving together the wisdom of taoist philosophy with the findings of quantum physics and the penetrating insight of Hahnemann, Mo provides a twenty-first century rendering of the timeless principles on which successful homoeopathic practice is based.

Whilst this book arose out of Mo's personal struggle to reconcile theoretical learning with the all too harsh reality of earning a living as a homoeopath, its message is a timely reminder for all of us. To practise authentically, we have to be willing to think for ourselves and have the courage of our own convictions, not someone else's. I can think of no better way to honour the spirit of Hahnemann's magnificent gift to humanity.

Ian Watson

Introduction

When I graduated I was a highflying 'classical homoeopath' ...and then I crashed! I began to realise that much of what I had understood was not helping me to earn a living for my family. I had learnt that all disease began in the mind, that I could only prescribe on mental and emotional symptoms (certainly not on 'physicals!') and that there was one remedy, the simillimum, which would cure the patient of everything, and be the only remedy he would ever need. I had understood that if I didn't find this 'right' remedy then I would give the 'wrong' one and the patient would 'prove it'. If I got the 'right' remedy but the 'wrong' potency then the patient might die, have a massive aggravation, or 'prove it'. If I got the 'right' remedy in the 'right' potency then the patient would get better according to the 'law of cure', if not then I would have 'suppressed' my patient and that was a very bad thing. If my patient broke her leg I could not prescribe even Arnica because it 'might interfere with deep-seated chronic constitutional treatment' (which would always end with a psoric eruption). People could only be treated if they came off all drugs and stopped drinking coffee. If my patient dared to clean her teeth with ordinary toothpaste then all my good work would be undone!

Suddenly I realised that this was not the kind of medicine that I wanted to practise. Soon afterwards I stumbled into an apprenticeship with Ken Metson (who used to see 20 to 30 patients per day) and began to break 'the rules'. What I discovered was a robust, simple, patient-friendly and effective system of medicine through which I could earn my living and contribute to my culture in a way that made sense to me. The fear of getting it 'wrong' was replaced by a quiet confidence...and people got better!

I was pleased, and a little uneasy. I studied hard yet deep down I was not sure enough that what I was doing and seeing was supported philosophically. Then, in 1997, came the second turning point. I began to study the *Organon of the Medical Art* as translated by Steven Decker and edited by Wenda Brewster O'Reilly (with a glossary!) Whilst it was obviously familiar to me, having studied other translations, it also seemed 'new' somehow. After a while I began to 'get it'. After a year or two Hahnemann's multi-dimensional model of a human being seemed to literally rise up out of the pages and inspire me. I persevered, I looked again at *The Chronic Diseases*, and philosophy and practice came closer and closer together.

What I have found the most difficult to do is to think 'outside the box' of classical Kentian thought. Kent was a genius **and** perhaps we haven't paid enough attention to Hahnemann. I certainly hadn't been able to until the 'new' translation.

This book represents my current understanding based on his teaching and what I have experienced in only fifteen years of practice. I feel compelled to write by a force, which I recognise as 'Ancestor'. It is filtered through a nature essentially Taoist and poetic, for which I make no apology. I write for my own clarification and I write for the new student, whom I will refer to as 'you'. I have included many quotes from Hahnemann because I want you to 'hear his voice'. I am not a scholar and this is not complete, it is minimal. You do not have to agree with anything written here, I only hope that it may dynamize and refresh your studies.

Homoeopathic medicine is a rational system of medicine based upon sound principles. Its practise is an art; beautiful, profound and simple. It is not a spiritual path or way to enlightenment, although it enhances and enriches such ways. It is '*an entirely simple medical art*'. It can be hard work, '*a very cogitative, laborious, arduous business. However, it fully restores the patient to health in a short time and without ailment so it becomes a curative and blessed business*' (*Organon* preface).

I can only encourage you to read Hahnemann and think. Think for yourself and then plunge into the stream of experience, and then think some more! In this way, I feel sure that your practice will become '*a curative and blessed business*'.

Making Your Own Experience

Reading this will be your experience as writing it has been mine. I hope it will be as clarifying and useful. All quotes in italics are from Dr Samuel Hahnemann and most are referenced. They are generally taken from:

1. *Organon of the Medical Art* (edited and annotated by Wenda Brewster O'Reilly Ph.D. and based on a translation by Steven Decker: adapted from the sixth edition of the *Organon der Heilkunst* completed by Samuel Hahnemann in 1842), Birdcage Books, Palo Alto, California, 1996. Quotes are denoted by aphorism number (Aph. 1), aphorism and footnote number (Aph. 1, fn. 1), or by introduction and page number (Intro. 8). Quotes taken from the glossary are denoted by the letter G followed by the page number (G 363).

2. *The Chronic Diseases - Their Peculiar Nature and Their Homoeopathic Cure* (theoretical part; completed by Samuel Hahnemann in 1838), B. Jain Publishers (P) Ltd., New Delhi, 2005. CD and page number denotes quotes (CD 35). Note: page numbers will differ in earlier editions.

I have chosen to work with the present tense of 'write'; for example, 'Hahnemann writes'. I know that he 'wrote' in the past but the present is where he continues to inspire me and 'writes' keeps it more alive and relevant for me. I have also chosen to write of the third person generally as 'he, him, and his'. With fullest respect for the Feminine, I am a man and my experience is masculine. The chapters are arranged in an order that makes sense to me. Feel free to read them as you will and then re-arrange or re-write them for yourself, according to your own sense. Most quotes are referenced and most chapters have a list of resources for your further exploration.

I hope that you will be encouraged to fill the spaces within the book with your own thoughts and questions. I would also strongly encourage you to read this alongside your readings of Hahnemann, Kent *et al.*

It is my intention to follow this book with another: *Medicine Flows: Homoeopathic Practice.* This will continue some of the explorations begun here in 'The Dynamic Practitioner', 'Case Taking' and 'Case Analysis'.

Make your own experience:
'No Guru, no method, no teacher.' (1)

References

1. Van Morrison. *No Guru, No Method, No Teacher.* Polydor, 1986.

Resources

1. James Tyler Kent. *Lectures on Homoeopathic Philosophy.* B. Jain Publishers (P) Ltd., New Delhi, 1987.
2. George Vithoulkas. *The Science of Homeopathy.* B. Jain Publishers (P) Ltd., New Delhi, 1980.
3. George Vithoulkas. *New Model for Health and Disease.* Health and Habitat and North Atlantic Books, 1991.
4. Stuart Close. *The Genius of Homeopathy.* B. Jain Publishers (P) Ltd., New Delhi, 1993.
5. Herbert A. Roberts. *The Principles and Art of Cure by Homoeopathy.* B. Jain Publishers (P) Ltd., New Delhi, 1985.
6. T. P. Paschero. *Homoeopathy.* Beaconsfield Publishers Ltd., U.K., 2000.
7. Francisco Xavier Eizayaga. *Treatise on Homoeopathic Medicine.* Ediciones Marcel, Buenos Aires, 1991.

1

Part One : The World

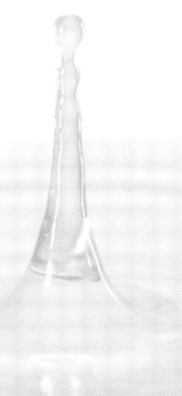

Life

In the study and practice of medicine I am working with live human beings, people who are in life, of life. My work is to help preserve life and improve the quality of life. In acute instances my work takes me to the edge of life…. and death.

Life! The great mystery, an awesome intangible. We all know it so well and yet we cannot grasp it, see it, measure it. We can only marvel at the range and complexity of the phenomena that it produces. We can only appreciate each other as individual expressions of this Life.

Being an intangible, life is difficult to define and almost impossible to hold in the net of words. A Standard English dictionary will suggest the following: **Life:** *The state or quality that distinguishes living beings or organisms from dead ones, and from inorganic matter; characterised by metabolism, growth, and the ability to reproduce and respond to stimuli.*

Metabolising, growing, reproducing, responding are all 'doing' words denoting activity and implying that living is the dynamic process of Life. Many dictionaries add the related adjective, 'animate'. **Animate:** *To give life to or cause to come alive: enliven. From Anima: breath or spirit.* **Spirit:** *The force or principle of life that animates the body of living things.*

The Greek word for life is *bios* from which we have derived bio, which indicates life or living organisms.

It seems clear to me that any study of living organisms (including biology and medicine) must acknowledge, find a place for, and work with, the force or principle of life. If not, then it is clear that these studies and disciplines should be using a different terminology!

One of the things I love about Life is its elusive nature, the way that it won't be pinned down or boxed. It has always seemed to me to be too full of wiggles and curves, giggles and paradox, to be grasped by left-brain linear thinking.

'The force that through the green fuse drives the flower.'

Dylan Thomas

In the study and practice of medicine I am working with the energy of Life!

Dynamic Medicine

The mainstream medical model is essentially molecular (concerning molecules) and is largely based upon 'Newtonian physics' (Newton died in 1727). The homoeopathic medical model is essentially dynamic (concerning energy or forces that produce motion) and relates well to 'quantum physics' (established by the mid-1920's).

The molecular model is both elegant and extremely useful. The dynamic model takes nothing away from this, it simply adds something. Energy. It takes notice of the force that moves molecules, the force which animates or enlivens the body, that force which leaves the body in the process of dying, the force whose presence enables us to distinguish between a living person and a corpse. Mainstream medicine is materialistic, relating to matter. Homoeopathic medicine is dynamic, relating to energy. Einstein famously wrote: 'We may therefore regard matter as being constituted by the regions of space in which the field is extremely intense... There is no place in this new kind of physics both for the field and matter, for the field is the only reality.' (1)

Essentially this 'field' refers to the infinite sea of energy that underlies all reality. Matter, however solid, is only a dense form of energy.

This 'new physics' does not seem to inform mainstream medical thinking or practice, at least not in the way in which it infuses homoeopathy and much of what I would call 'holistic medicine'. Einstein could be re-written: 'There is no place in this new kind of medicine for both the field and matter, for the field is the only reality.'

At the present time this energy, this force, cannot be measured and so is ignored by orthodox thinking. This is a limitation. To try to 'prove' a dynamic model within the confines of a material model is difficult, if not impossible.

Meanwhile, sickness on this planet is not decreasing...AT ALL! Suffering humanity needs all the help it can get. We could work together.

Throughout this work the terms 'energy' and 'matter' will be used to refer to either 'pole' within the field. The understanding is that matter is a dense form of energy.

References
1. Fritjof Capra. *The Tao of Physics*. Flamingo, London, 1983, p. 233.

The Field

The 'new physics' suggests that the universe is one unified and infinite field of energy, a dynamic and multi-dimensional web through which all things are connected. It also suggests that living beings constantly exchange energy and information with this inexhaustible quantum field. Every thing in existence is made from the same basic 'stuff', energy. I like the ancient Persian thought:

> 'Rock is Life asleep,
> Plant is Life dreaming,
> Animal is Life awake,
> Man is Life becoming conscious of itself.' (1)

From this I choose to call the basic 'stuff' life, or '*life force*'. Rock then is this life force organised and expressed in one way, whilst I am life force organised and expressed in another. I understand that rock is not 'alive' according to standard criteria. From a more universal, and inclusive, perspective it is alive because it is energetic and has an organising principle that maintains it as itself. Perhaps it is only a matter of the degree of alive-ness.

Each living thing is constituted when energies come together somewhere in the field and then emerge from it, as one. Such a coalescence is a fusing or blending of energetic vibrations with the purpose of increasing or nourishing an aspect of Life. Because 'energy and matter', 'particle and wave', 'life and death', 'psyche and soma' etc. express the perceived polarity within this unified field, the primary dynamic motion or movement of existence would seem to be a pulsation: a rhythmic contraction and expansion, a one to the other-ness.

Taoism expresses this idea beautifully in the T'ai-chi T'u or Diagram of the Supreme Ultimate (Figure 1).

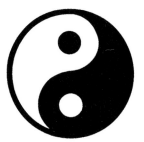

Figure 1 - T'ai Chi Tu

This simple rhythm creates waves.

References
1. Something I read many years ago, source unknown.

Resources
1. Lao Tsu. *The Tao Te Ching*. Many translations.
2. Almost anything written by Alan Watts.
3. Lynne McTaggart. The Field – *The Quest for the Secret Force of the Universe*. HarperCollins Publishers Ltd., 2001.

2

Part Two : The Human

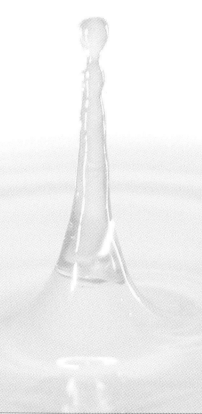

Medicine Flows

Organism

In the relative darkness of my mother's womb a single egg and a single sperm come together to form a single cell, the first molecular evidence of a new individual.... me! This becomes my experience-packed life, still living itself as vibrantly as possible over fifty years later. How does this happen?

A fresh new fusion of energy emerges from the field and begins to pulsate as an individual dynamic entity. Over time (whatever that may be) this entity exchanges energy and information with the field and organises itself into one life in the great ocean of human being. How is this organised?

Human being is an activity. The human organism is an extraordinarily complex organic system. All the integral parts are organised into a structured whole and their functions are harmoniously coordinated. The thinking, feeling, willing, healthy human organism is a phenomenon, unique and miraculous. As much as we know about it, we could acknowledge that we do not know. There is still mystery here. Just the level of orchestration of the trillions of multi-functioning cells and their intra-cellular complexity is beyond our comprehension. The fact that in one year's time 98% of the atoms in my body will have changed and yet I will still be recognizable as me, is an everyday miracle. How does that happen? What is it that keeps me together as me? Again, what is it that coordinates, orchestrates, organises?

The root of organise, organism, organelle, organic is **organ**. This derives from the Greek word **Organon**, meaning tool or instrument.

So, an organ is a tool or instrument with which/through which work can be done or accomplished. There is a usefulness here as well as a musicality. The biological principle that 'function creates and develops the organ' implies that activity, and thereby life force, creates and develops the organ. When billions of organelles and a number of organs are organised into an organism whose organic structure and functioning is harmoniously coordinated, how much more useful is the greater whole! How appropriate are such terms as 'harmonious' and 'orchestration'! The point is that the language we use in reference to the human organism implies a dynamic, implies energy, implies and involves the life force or life principle. It also hints at a certain usefulness and musicality. This is common to all medical practice.

Within homoeopathic medicine the word 'organon' strikes a particular note or chord. Dr Samuel Hahnemann titled his masterwork the *Organon of the Medical Art*. Here, 'organon' is taken to mean 'an instrument of thought or knowledge, especially a set of principles for use in scientific or philosophical investigation'.

Within the *Organon* (as clarified by Decker and O'Reilly) Hahnemann expands upon the dynamic nature of the human organism and presents a dynamic model of health, sickness and cure. He also takes up the idea of instrument, from both a musical and utilitarian perspective. The following chapter represents my understanding and individual expression of that.

The Instrument

'*In the healthy human state, the spirit-like life force (autocracy) that enlivens the material organism as dynamis, governs without restriction and keeps all parts of the organism in admirable, harmonious, vital operation, as regards both feelings and functions, so that our indwelling, rational spirit can freely avail itself of this living, healthy instrument for the higher purposes of our existence.*' (Aph. 9)

The human organism exists and happens in the space-time continuum and may be viewed as an instrument, an instrument of life, having some purpose in life. Each human organism exists and happens within the greater organism of the human race and life on Earth. Each individual exists and happens as a bio-field within the greater field of energy.

Within the individual, the life force which '*en-livens*' or animates the material organism is governed or organised by the '*life principle*' or '*dynamis*' ('*wesen*: essence: nature: entity') (G 361). This is a 'dynamic self-subsisting presence' which is 'not material and has no mass' (G 362). The dynamis orders the instinctual vital operation of the organism through direction of the life force.

It is as if the dynamis is somehow plugged into the field and gathers energy and information from it into itself. Over time the dynamis organises a whole human experience. It moves molecules and organises the individual field into material, dynamic and psychical planes, levels or faculties.

All of these planes are dynamic in essence. All of them '*constitute a unity, although in thought we split this unity into…concepts in order to conceptualise it more easily*' (Aph. 15).

Unity means that every aspect of the life force is present in every other (perhaps like in a hologram) and that the energy flows or moves naturally from one plane to another. Each aspect or plane has its own differentiated quality, its own vibration, tone, frequency… or potency.

The material plane is the plane of the body. This is where the field is most dense. This is the plane of gross anatomy and gross pathology. This plane is organised from atoms and molecules into trillions of cells. These cells are further organised into tissues and systems with fully differentiated governing organs such as the brain and heart. The subtlest and most fluid aspects of the anatomy on this plane are the nervous, endocrine and immune systems. Gross anatomy relates more to structure whilst fluid anatomy relates more to function.

What I am calling the dynamic plane is the plane of the dynamis and the undifferentiated life force, the plane of animation. The field here is invisible and intangible, less dense and concrete, much more subtle and discrete, '*spirit-like*'. (In traditional Chinese medicine this life force is called 'chi' and moves along specific pathways called meridians.) The organising principle here is the dynamis, probably the most energetic and dynamic aspect of the organism because it is constantly organising and coordinating everything through the movement of instinctual life force.

Hahnemann writes of the '*sustentive power*' (Aph. 63) of the life force that, in health, maintains the organism in '*harmonious vital operation*'. It is this aspect that attempts to restore balance and heal wounds, to sustain health. The natural state of the life force is health and it is to the state of health that it will always attempt to return. He also writes of the generative power of the life force, involved in reproduction and the '*engenderment*' of disease (Intro. 37).

The 'psychical' plane is the plane of the psyche, the self, the most individual aspect of the whole human being. The field here may be the most subtle and discrete. It is the plane where consciousness arises and unconsciousness continues. The field is organised into three distinct faculties or '*almost spiritual, mental and emotional organs, which have never been reached, and are unreachable by any dissecting scalpel*' (Aph. 216).

The **Geist** (G 351): spirit; intellectual mind. The most subtle aspect, 'the faculty of pure intelligence in the human being, which is manifested through the operations of intellect and reason'. This gives rise to the intellectual kind of knowledge that Hahnemann refers to as '*wissen*'. This is, perhaps, that faculty which enables us to form more conscious connections with the greater sense of Life or Spirit outside of ourselves. The Geist is one of two 'supersensible presences that permeate the organism', the other being the dynamis. Together they represent the two poles of human being: intellect and instinct.

The **Gemüt** (G 305): emotional mind. This is an 'aesthetic faculty' and has to do with 'participative consciousness'. It gives us the ability to take in impressions and have responses to them, giving rise to the experiential kind of knowledge that Hahnemann refers to as '*kennen*'. The Gemüt may therefore be the '*almost spiritual organ*' of relationship (see Susceptibility), allowing feelings to be felt, held, or emoted and sensations to be experienced within the body.

The **Soul** (G 350): the 'intermediary between the spirit and the emotional mind'. Tradition suggests that soul occupies the centre of a human life where it is considered to be the seat of both the conscience and the will. The interaction between these three components of the psychical plane gives rise to thinking, feeling and willing within an individual (Figure 2).

Human being then is the result of the simultaneous integration of these three planes. Harmonious vital coordination and operation gives rise to a healthy human organism: an organism with an overall soundness (*Gesundheit*) of vibration or tone. Whilst each plane (or any aspect of each plane) may have its own vibration, note or tone at any one time, the most consistent, fundamental and general frequency of any individual will relate to its constitution or basic make-up. It also relates to the fundamental state of health, as expressed by the most consistently experienced and observable mental, emotional and physical characteristics over time.

When in tune '*this living healthy instrument*' may be used by the indwelling spirit for the greater good of the individual and his community.

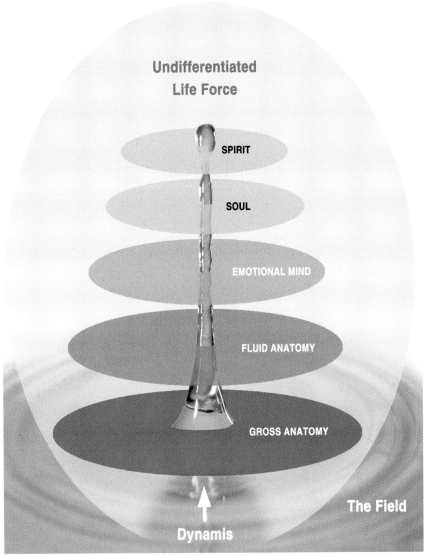

Figure 2: A diagrammatic representation of the levels of organisation within the human being.

It is clear to me that an invisible and intangible, differentiated, '*spirit-like*' and dynamic anatomy was implicit in Hahnemann's description of a human being.

To practise homoeopathic medicine a dynamic model is absolutely essential.

Notes

- Hahnemann worked with a dynamic model of human being that was more subtle and sophisticated than just '*vital force*'.
- As I understand it, the 'Seven Levels' model of Dr Rajan Sankaran (1) can easily be super-imposed upon the model of Hahnemann. I find this encouraging!

References

1. Personal notes made during a nine-day seminar with Dr Sankaran, Mumbai, India, January 2004.

Tunement

The healthy human organism is a dynamic instrument, an integrated and individual energetic entity with an overall fundamental resonant frequency, note, or tone. It is 'in tune' with itself and its environment, it has its own particular 'tunement'. Any disturbing influence or dynamic impingement upon the life force can induce a '*mistunement*', an alteration in this frequency or tone. The instrument is now 'out of tune', health has been altered to a disease state, and '*adverse sensations*' and '*irregular functions*' (symptoms) have been induced. Prolonged disturbance or continued mistunement may ultimate in tissue change or gross pathology. If accompanied by suppressions it may induce a more or less permanent '*attunement*' to disease (see Miasm).

Disturbance or mistunement is communicated through the dynamic plane. An ordering influence on the life force can also induce an alteration in the frequency or tone, a '*re-tunement*'. The characteristic tone has been restored, disease has been lifted to a healthy state, and '*harmonious vital operation*' has returned sensation and function to normal.

A medicinal potence, capable of inducing a similar, yet slightly increased mistunement in a healthy life force, appears to '*overtune*' (Aph. 68) the life force in the process of cure. This overtunement may be experienced by the organism as an aggravation of symptoms. The slightly over-tuned life force can no longer experience the similar natural mistunement, and this falls away, as it were. The stimulated life force then reacts against the medicinal potence in the process of '*re-tunement*'.

It is my understanding that the mechanism of mis-tuning and re-tuning is the same.

The work of the homoeopath is to re-tune, and then fine-tune the individual instrument. Tuning a musical instrument is an art, fine-tuning is a more subtle art. It comes down to having a 'good ear', or sense of attunement. This may be natural, or learned with experience. It is the same with the re-tunement of a human organism. Ultimately it is an art requiring a dynamic sense.

The work of the homoeopath is also to make sound suggestions as to how the organism may best be kept in tune.

Conversational Observation / Resonance Readings

Also - ♀1 positive word → meds ♀2 positive memory or association

♀2 → visible difference in person's face / body language (positive resonance)

Connection and Resonance

For the phenomenal organism to be able to grow, develop and experience itself it needs to enter into relationship with the surrounding field. For this to happen there first of all needs to be resonance. This means that there has to be a degree of dynamic similarity, affinity or sympathy between two 'bodies' before communication can take place.

Resonance is the 'sound' produced by a body vibrating in sympathy with a neighbour, two tuning forks for example. First there is sound and then there is re-sound. Essentially that sound is 'hello' and it means that there is a degree of recognition and relationship (of affinity or harmony). The more intense and clear the re-sound the greater the potential for intimate relationship. The quality of this relationship is important; it may be beneficial or it may be harmful. *In extremis* it may be fatal.

Put another way, the resonant frequency of two vibrating, pulsating entities needs to be similar if connection is to become more intimate. This is the phenomenon of attraction, of 'like attracting like'. This attraction can manifest at every level of dynamic organisation, from the sub-atomic to the purely spiritual. The greater the resonance, the greater the susceptibility to influence.

Sometimes a large number of dynamic instruments gather together with a common purpose or focus of attention (such as life force organised as festival or crowd). If the communication between them is clear then a particular quality of vibration or atmosphere is generated and there is a sense of connection, excitement and in-tunement. Often such an event is described as a 'resounding success'!

Underlying all sound and re-sound is the Great Sound with which all living things resonate.

 Eg   Healing groups harmoniously resonate

Susceptibility

The 'Germ Theory of Disease' maintains that many diseases are caused by the invasion of our system by microorganisms. Louis Pasteur, greatly involved in the formation of this theory, appeared to change his mind at the end of his life by declaring 'c'est le terrain!' By this he meant that, whilst the microbe has a part to play, it is the soil, the susceptibility of the person that is the key element.

It has always seemed to me that susceptibility is fundamental to the practice of all medicine. It becomes increasingly clear to me that susceptibility is also fundamental to the continuance and development of Life itself.

When discussing the power of dynamic influences ('*inimical potences*') to '*morbidly mistune*' the human life force, Hahnemann writes:

'*We become diseased by them only when our organism is just exactly and sufficiently disposed and laid open to be assailed* [by them], *and to be altered in its condition, mistuned and displaced into abnormal feelings and functions.*' (Aph. 31)

He then writes that '*the living human organism is far more disposed and inclined to allow itself to be aroused and have its condition differently tuned by medicinal powers*' than natural disease-causing influences (Aph. 33). In other translations of these aphorisms the word 'susceptible' is used. It seems to me that Hahnemann is describing a passivity, or receptivity, which can be '*aroused*' into activity or reactivity.

In all my other reading of the homoeopathic literature on susceptibility (notably Kent, Close, Roberts, Vithoulkas) I have found uncertainty and confusion. On the one hand there are ideas such as 'open-ness', 'vacuum', 'yielding'; on the other hand, 'the reaction of the organism to internal and external influences'. An aphorism from Kent has always moved me to think about this:

'Whatever a man is susceptible to, such he is, such is his quality.' (1)

This suggests to me that susceptibility is a fundamental attribute of human being. When I re-write this as: 'Whatever a man yields to, such he is, such is his quality', it seems incomplete. Also: 'Whatever a man reacts to, such he is, such is his quality', does not quite hold his is-ness, his quality.

Whatever a man yields to, **and** how he reacts to it, **that** tells me much more about his nature, his is-ness, or quality. In fact these together tell me pretty much everything there is to know about him, apart from his appearance.

Susceptibility relates to the dynamic state of the organism. It is a quality or aspect of the life force that enables it to yield to a dynamic influence and then to respond to the impression made upon it by that influence. To put it in a slightly different way, it is the ability of the organism to receive information/stimuli and then to respond. The more appropriate the response to the situation the greater the health of the organism.

As human beings it is in our nature to grow, to evolve, to fulfil our potential. To do this we need to be able to change. We need to be able to take up, to be influenced, to be aroused. We all have our needs, desires, vacuums, gaps, wounds and yearnings. They exist on every level and because of them we attract to us, or seek out, the things that we lack, those things that can help us to move towards wholeness. We need things such as food, shelter, work, relationship and disease to influence us in the direction of completeness, one-ness. If we cannot yield to influence then we cannot change.

In the *Tao Te Ching* the word influence (influx, inflowance) comes from the Chinese word Ch'I that means 'breath' or 'vital force'. This reminds me of the dynamic nature of the process.

The life force yields to the dynamic influence and allows it to make its impression. The impressed life force is thereby altered or differently tuned. A change in tone or note means that resonance has ceased and the individual is no longer open to the influence. Resistance has been met and immunity has been established. This different tunement may be experienced by the individual as a benefit, or as a symptom.

Being open to influence is essential for change, growth and maturation. Being able to offer resistance to an influence is essential to the preservation of individuality. Resistance is about limit; it is the universal way of saying 'That's enough!' If there were no resistance there could be no individuality, boundaries would be continually breached. Nothing really is, nothing can be unique, unless it has limit. Even the degree of resistance, and the time taken to reach the point of resistance, is individual. At this point or place of resistance the influence has made its fullest impression on the life force.

'Specifically, impressions are made upon the life force organised in the emotional mind (the Gemüt) which is the aesthetic faculty.' (G 316)

It is interesting to note that in most dictionaries the word 'impression' has a strong emotional bias, as in 'she's so impressionable', and 'artistic impression'. It makes sense that feelings, experienced in the emotional mind, and sensations, experienced in the body mind (as somatic feelings) are the different poles of this 'aesthetic faculty'. This may form the basis for the 'felt sense' through which we experience others.

We need the ability to respond to impressions, to react to changes, to adapt, or we may die. Once we have filled our belly we need to digest and assimilate. Once we have read enough homoeopathic philosophy we need to reflect and integrate. Once we have received a blow on any level we need to 'come back'. An organism can only 'take on board' just so much of anything at any one time before there is a natural resistance, and then reaction. This whole process is explained in aphorism 63 of the *Organon*:

*'Each life-impinging potence, each medicine, alters the tuning of the life force more or less and arouses a certain alteration of a person's condition for a longer or shorter time. This is termed the **initial action**. While the initial action is a product of*

both the medicinal energy and the life force, it **belongs more** *to the impinging potence [of the medicine]. Our life force strives to oppose this impinging action with its own energy. This back-action belongs to our sustentive power of life and is an automatic function of it, called the* **after-action** *or* **counter-action.'**

The dynamic word here is '*impinging*'; this means 'to have superficial contact with something, followed by a thrusting, driving or penetration into it' (G 316). This suggests to me a manner of influencing that is essentially masculine, a stimulus for change that is pointed, penetrating and sudden. Influencing through 'inflowance' suggests a process that is essentially feminine, rounded, suffusing and gradual. I wonder if more '*spirit-like*' agents, such as a viral dynamis, a stinging rebuke, a dynamised medicine, influence in a masculine way whereas more material agents such as poisons, upbringing and environment, or herbal remedies, influence in a feminine way? This feminine/masculine aspect is reinforced in aphorism 64:

'*...during the initial action.....our life force' (organised in its generative aspect) 'appears to comport itself only conceptively (receptively, passively as it were) and appears as if it were forced to allow the impressions of the artificial potence impinging from without to occur in itself...*'

In his preface to the fourth volume of *The Chronic Diseases* (and also in his introduction to the *Organon*) Hahnemann is clear that '*un-assisted*', the life force is no match for the hostile influences that cause disease, i.e. '*our vital force hardly opposes an equal opposition*' (CD xxi).

'Action and reaction are equal and opposite' is a law of physics (2) that does not seem to apply so well on the dynamic planes of Bio. If it were so then we would always return to health naturally and would have no need of the medicine. The reason we don't may be due to the individual nature of susceptibility. Without reaction, individuality would be undermined. The timing and quality of an organism's reaction to influence is an expression of this individuality. This is demonstrated in the process of learning which involves at least two aspects: the reception of and engagement with new material and then, the response to it.

Again, the first part of this process is relatively passive whilst the second is more active. This process seems to be a fundamental aspect of the dynamics of relationship. This is easy to understand with regards to inter-personal relationship, which is entirely based on reacting to impressions. 'Our eyes met across a crowded dance floor. I smiled, she smiled (resonance); I asked her to dance and she said 'Yes!'

In a similar way I could say that I am in relationship with you, because you are reading my words, now. *Medicine Flows* was my 'hello' to which you responded with 'Hello, what's this then?' It seems that enough of an impression was created within for you to have at least opened the book and turned to this page. Will you yield some more?

The process can be written in a number of ways:

Resonance: open-ness; influence; impression; resistance; reaction.
Chime: yield; inflow; impress; limit; return.

The passive and active aspects of this process seem to be mutually arising. That is to say they give rise to one another, complement one another.

> 'Returning is the motion of the Tao.
> Yielding is the way of the Tao.'
>
> *Lao Tsu*

The idea of susceptibility offered here incorporates yielding and returning and suggests that, perhaps, they may form a 'functional polarity' (G 311) whose common functioning principle is relationship. It is difficult to ignore a natural polarity here:

Passive-Active
Open-Closed
Empty-Full
Action-Reaction
Ebb-Flow
Ignorance-Knowledge

This polarity involves movement, a one-to-the-other-ness, a rhythm. This rhythm is natural, unforced, easy; it happens of itself like breathing, like antibody production.

Susceptibility may be seen as an aspect of the life force or dynamis which is fundamental to the movement between sickness and health, the process of both contagion and cure, the relationship between one and the other. This relationship may manifest as a dance with a partner, a dance with an idea, or a dance with a virus. Further, I offer that susceptibility may also be seen as an aspect of the greater Life Force or Dynamis and the movement between life and death, energy and matter, psyche and soma: the fluid mechanism behind change.

> First there is the One.
> Then there is the one and the other.
> Then the movement between the two,
> The relationship
> Which creates all things.

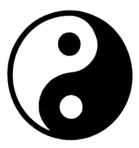

There is a sense of fluidity here, of flexibility and adaptation.

> 'A man is born gentle and weak, at his death he is hard and stiff.
> Green plants are tender and filled with sap, at their death they are
> withered and dry.
> Therefore the stiff and unbending is the disciple of death
> The gentle and yielding is the disciple of life.'

Lao Tsu

As a practitioner I want to preserve this quality, to preserve life and growth, to encourage the fulfilment of potential. I want the people I work with to be open to life and yet able to respond to it appropriately. I need to be able to alter their susceptibility with the medicines and words that I administer.

As examples: an individual may be too open ('overly impressionable to every external influence') and respond well to Phosphorus. He may be too closed ('walled off') and benefit from Natrum muriaticum. An overly reactive Nux vomica state is often described as 'a violin string about to snap' ('very irritable and sensitive to all impressions') whilst homoeopathic Opium can be very helpful to someone manifesting 'extreme placidity' or 'lack of vital reaction'.

'This power to modify susceptibility is the basis of the art of the physician.' (3)

I am suggesting that susceptibility exists at every level of the organism, whether the life force is organised as organ, constitution, or intellect. It will also exist at every level of the greater whole, whether the Life Force is organised as family, city, race or planet.

Factors which give rise to or modify susceptibility include inheritance (miasmatic or genetic) constitution, age, lifestyle and environment, upbringing and life experience, pathology, treatment etc.

'Without susceptibility all our efforts to cure are in vain.' (4)

Notes
- ☉ I have chosen to use the word susceptibility to cover the whole dynamic process of yielding to an influence and then responding to the impression made by it upon the life force.
- ☉ Susceptibility is fundamental to being alive, not just to becoming diseased.
- ☉ Potences, whether healthful or harmful, impinge upon the life force.

The impression of a potence appears to be made specifically upon the life force organised as the Gemüt. This impression is likely to be first experienced by the organism as either a feeling or a sensation: 'the vital sensation' (5). There is not necessarily a mental or emotional symptom.

References

1. James Tyler Kent. *New Remedies, Clinical Cases; Lesser Writings, Aphorisms and Precepts.* Ehrhart and Karl, Chicago, 1926, aphorism 269.
2. Sir Isaac Newton. *Principia Mathematica Philosophiae Naturalis.* 1686. ("For every action there is an equal and opposite reaction.")
3. Stuart Close. *The Genius of Homeopathy.* B. Jain Publishers (P) Ltd., New Delhi, 1993, p. 77.
4. Stuart Close. *The Genius of Homeopathy.* B. Jain Publishers (P) Ltd., New Delhi, 1993, p. 79.
5. Personal notes taken during a nine-day seminar with Dr Rajan Sankaran, Mumbai, 2004.

Suppression

Sometimes the life force is prevented from flowing, acting, or reacting according to its nature. This is not always harmful. A blocked stream can find another way to the sea; a growing child needs a 'no' occasionally, needs boundaries within which to grow safely. Adaptation and evolution may result in benefits. Often, however, this prevention or suppression can damage the organism.

To suppress is to restrain, to go against the natural flow. Feelings, for example, arise naturally and spontaneously move or emote in the process of self-expression. If we repress or deny these emotions then we go against the natural flow of our lives, we live the life that is not our true one and we pay the price.

In terms of medicine, orthodox drugs, by their very names, are intentionally anti-flow agents. Examples include anti-depressants, anti-inflammatories and anti-biotics. These anti-flow agents may save lives in the short term but are almost always harmful in the long term.

Homoeopathic medicine works and moves with the life force. A truly homoeopathic medicine promotes and encourages flow and will not suppress. 'Homoeopathic suppression' makes no sense, does it? More experienced practitioners than I have reported such a phenomenon yet it is not part of my experience.

Constitution

'The constitution is that which is.' (1)

This term relates to the way in which the human being is composed, how all the separable aspects hang together or relate at a fundamental level. It refers to a person's basic structure and way of functioning in health. The composition, the being-together-ness of each human, in terms of structure and function, has an individual dynamic quality. This quality manifests as an overall and relative soundness, a characteristic tone of the life force. We use terms such as 'robust constitution' or 'delicate constitution' to describe the quality of this basic make-up. It represents the most rounded expression of the dynamis in the state of health. It encompasses the healthy characteristics and susceptibilities of the individual, characteristics of personality, body-type, food desires and aversions and general modalities.

Over a lifetime filled with work and all the various stresses of human being, the constitution will begin to break down, to de-compose, as part of the spiral towards death. Then we use phrases such as 'worn out' or 'broken down' constitutions.

Various writers have attempted to describe and differentiate between 'constitutional types' and to describe homoeopathic medicines that are related to, or are expressions of, these types. Léon Vannier (1), extending the work of Nebel (2) described the Carbonic, Phosphoric and Fluoric constitutions. Von Grauvogl (3) wrote of the Hydrogenoid, Oxygenoid, and Carbo-Nitrogenoid types. Eizayaga (4) suggests that if we are to find a medicine for the constitution then 'we shall be limited to prescribe from 12-14 medicines'. He writes of 'characterologic features' that are not real symptoms, such as industrious, cheerful, calm, courageous etc. None of these are pathological; none can be treated much less cured! We prescribe on these characteristics 'to prevent future ailments'. Constitutional treatment is to do with sustaining and maintaining the basic level of health.

In aphorism 6 Hahnemann writes that we are to take notice only of '*the deviations from the former healthy state*'. Hahnemann treated diseases, not the healthy state; Hahnemann did not prescribe constitutionally.

In practice I find it quite useful to have a sense of a patient's basic quality or constitution, if it can be discerned, and whether or not it relates to a medicinal 'picture'. Is he fundamentally strong, weak, or broken down? This can be helpful in choosing potency for example.

Notes

○ If you are going to use the term 'constitution', be clear what you mean.

References

1. Léon Vannier. *Typology in Homoeopathy*. Beaconsfield Publishers Ltd., 1992, p. 1.
2. Jacques Jouanny. *The Essentials of Homeopathic Therapeutics*. Boiron S.A. France, 1993, p. 65.
3. John H. Clarke. *Constitutional Medicine*. B. Jain Publishers (P) Ltd., 1995.
4. Francisco Xavier Eizayaga. *Treatise on Homoeopathic Medicine*. Ediciones Marcel, Buenos Aires, 1991, p. 282.

Health

Hahnemann uses the German word 'Gesundheit' meaning soundness. This suggests something free from damage or decay, something unbroken, whole, complete, or solid. Being 'sound asleep' is to sleep deeply, peacefully, without disturbance; such sleep is naturally restorative. We have the expression 'as sound as a bell', again suggesting something unbroken, well made, and also something that produces a clear sound, a musical note or tone. This reminds me of *'the living, healthy instrument'*.

It would seem that the stronger the tone the greater the harmony between all parts of the instrument. The clearer the note the greater the resonance with a neighbouring instrument, and the more musical and harmonious the sound produced between them. This is the beginning of dynamic relationship, of vibrant community. It may also be the beginning of symphony!

The quality of health is ease and freedom, freedom from constriction, resistance and pain. With no friction movement is easy, its expression fulfilling and stillness its natural complement. In health there is harmony, the tone is strong, the note is clear, the sound is music, the movement is an easy rhythm and the direction is upward and outward into relationship, into the re-sound dance which is so necessary for the experience and knowing of self.

In health I am in tune with myself, and with my world. I am fully present. All is 'well' (from Old Norse meaning good). 'Health' comes from Old English 'hael', meaning whole; complete; sound.

Where there is wholeness then, sooner or later there will be broken-ness too. Well becomes 'ill' (from Old Norse meaning bad, harm, pain) and ease (freedom from discomfort, anxiety, poverty) becomes dis-ease (apart from freedom). The instrument is out of tune, both with itself and with its neighbours. Dissonance prevails, cacophony results.

The quality of dis-ease is constriction, resistance and pain. With friction, movement hurts, stillness agitates and expression is tuned to suffering. In sickness there is disharmony, the tone is weak, the note is distorted, the sound is noise, the movement is a jerky dis-rhythm and the direction is inward and downward, 'under the doctor', 'into the hospital' and into the disconnection which is also so necessary for the experience and knowing of self.

Health and dis-ease are mutually arising, they are in complementary relationship with one another. One cannot exist without the other, and the state of one is always relative to the other. Any attempt to 'eradicate disease' is not mindful of this and so is futile, stupid and dangerous.

3

Part Three : Disease

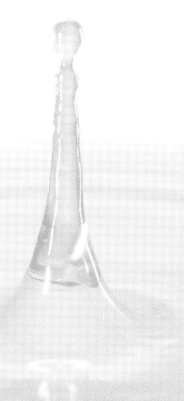

Disease

'*When a person falls ill, it is initially only this spirit-like life force (life principle) everywhere present in the organism that is mistuned through the dynamic influence of a morbific agent inimical to life. Only the life principle, mistuned to such abnormality, can impart to the organism the adverse sensations and induce in the organism the irregular functions that we call disease.*' (Aph. 11)

The dynamis of a disease-inducing agent (potence) impinges upon the dynamis of a susceptible organism and impresses itself there. Primary symptoms are produced. The dynamis then opposes the agent's action with its own energy and secondary symptoms may be produced. In this diseased state the life force instinctively does what it can to preserve life and restore health. *In extremis* it '*sacrifices and destroys suffering parts in order to save the rest*' (Intro. p. 28, fn. 21).

The relationship between the disease potence and the dynamis of the organism forms a separate dynamis, the disease. This results from a mistunement of the dynamis by the potence and is expressed through signs and symptoms, changes in sensation and function, changes in state, condition and appearance.

The numerical sum of all the symptoms is the '*totality of symptoms*'; it is quantitative. The characteristic symptoms, which hang together and express the individual nature of the disease dynamis, form the '*symptom complex*' (Aph. 16). This is qualitative and is organised by the dynamis. (Hahnemann seems to use '*symptom complex*' and '*totality of symptoms*' interchangeably; this is clarified in G 355.) There are three basic types of disease-causing agent or potence:

Infective: such as a virulent microbe.
Affective: such as an insult or a false belief.
Toxic: such as a poison or drug.

Another major kind of influence would seem to be a lack of certain energies essential for life, such as food, warmth, affection etc.

There is the idea that 'there are no diseases only sick people' from which it follows that 'we don't treat diseases we treat people'. This is only partially true. If disease is a mistunement of the life force and the homoeopath works with medicines to re-tune that life force, to return it to its healthiest state, then the homoeopath treats disease. The disease, however, is dynamic, consists of more than symptoms and can only arise within a living organism.

Any '*deviation from the former healthy state*' (Aph. 6) is a diseased state. Hahnemann teaches us to treat the disease '*in its entirety*', that is to treat both the dynamic mistunement **and** its expression through symptoms. For Hahnemann, a disease is a definite entity with its own dynamis and character. This relates to the idea of the '*genus epidemicus*' (G 312), a dynamic symptom complex observable in the collective, in a group of people. Many times I have seen people who have benefited greatly from medicines such as Lycopodium, Natrum muriaticum etc. produce similar symptoms in an epidemic of 'that bug that's going around'. Together they produce a collective symptom complex due to the influence of the 'bug' dynamis, and they all then respond to a medicinal dynamis such as Arnica or Radium bromide. Once restored, they may then benefit from 'constitutional treatment' to keep them well.

There is a dynamic process involved in the creation of disease. The healthy person is at ease; he is energetically sound (albeit with inherited or individual tendencies, pre-dispositions to disease - see Miasm). Because Life is dynamic, there will be times when he falls apart from ease and enters the state of dis-ease. This will be due to a change in his life force, a change in his personal bio-field of energy, as a result of being alive on a planet. These changes can be brought about by stress, work, relationships etc. This state is solely dynamic and relates to susceptibility. The patient may feel 'unwell' in a vague sense, a kind of pro-dromal period, and then a disease state may be generated with changes in normal sensation and function. In certain situations disease may move on to pathology, that is to changes in tissue structure. The end result of the diseasing process may be gross pathology, or marked tissue change, and death.

Health and disease are mutually arising and may be seen as relative states of ease. Maybe all one can ever comment on is the direction the life process seems to be moving in, whether it is easing or diseasing.

EASE: DIS-EASE: DISEASE: PATHOLOGY: GROSS-PATHOLOGY
>---------Diseasing, embodying, enburdening, separating
<---------Easing, enlightening, unifying

In the assessment of the relative health of an individual the homoeopath has to consider that individual's state, condition and appearance.

The state of an individual refers specifically to the quality of the psychical plane at the time, and is primarily perceived through his behaviour. State is a qualitative phenomenon that can only be discerned through the aware participation of the homoeopath. A diseased state is characterised by an altered or false sense of reality, a delusion. An example might be: 'I'm fine, I don't need any help', when the patient clearly does.

Behaviour is also influenced by the emotional state, the quality of the Gemüt. The '*pre-eminent importance of the emotional state holds good to such an extent that the patient's emotional state often tips the scales in the selection of the homoeopathic remedy*' (Aph. 211). An example might be the patient shouting and cursing angrily and out of proportion to the situation.

Condition refers to feelings, functions and sensations and so relates more to the body-mind, the emotional mind within the body. A diseased condition is characterised by negative feelings, malfunctions and uncomfortable sensations. Hahnemann sometimes uses the term '*condition-state*' (G 296) which implies that they are inter-related aspects of the larger dynamic of human being.

Appearance speaks for itself and includes objective signs of disease.

So, disease is a dynamic mistunement of the life force. This manifests through changes in state, condition and appearance as expressed through signs and symptoms. These are experienced by the patient and observed or perceived by those around him. A symptom is a subjective indication of disease, one experienced by the patient as 'I feel', or by the practitioner as 'I sense'. A sign is an objective indication of disease and includes diagnostic test data as well as clinical observations.

Reading the *Organon* it becomes clear to me that Hahnemann did not advocate prescribing upon the symptoms alone. The homoeopath perceives and considers only:

'*the deviations from the former healthy state of the now sick patient*' (Aph.6);
'*the alterations in the condition of body and soul, disease signs, befallments, symptoms*' (Aph. 6);
'*any contingent miasm*' and the '*attendant circumstances*' (Aph. 7);
'*the totality of symptoms for the disease case, with regard for the originating cause (when it is known) and for the accessory circumstances*' (Aph. 24).

All of these aspects of disease are contained within the totality of symptoms. '*All these perceptible signs represent the disease in its* **entire** *extent*' (my emphasis); '*that is* **together**' (me again) '*they form the true and only conceivable gestalt of the disease*' (Aph. 6).

'*Befallments*' includes the phenomena of accidents and incidents in the life of the person. This insists upon a consideration of potential cause, the 'Never Been Well Since'. This suggests that a disease '*in its entirety*' is made up of the cause, the mistunement, and the expression of that.

Dr Burnett comments beautifully: 'The contention that the disease is **all** expressed in the symptoms is one to which I cannot assent'.

'It is **not enough** to cover the totality of symptoms; for when this has been done we are only half way, we have then to ask these questions: what is the real nature, the natural history, the pathology of the malady under consideration? What caused it? Is the cause still there or has it gone? Is the drug chosen capable of producing a real disease like the one before us? In fact: is it **really** homoeopathic to the morbid process, reaching from beginning to end? If **not**, we are **on the wrong scent if we are to really cure and not merely palliate**.' (1)

Hahnemann writes that '*after the lifting of all the symptoms of the disease and of the entire complex of perceptible befallments*' (Aph. 8) only health can remain.

This '*entire complex*' is located within the ambient (G 285). This is the field or aura within and around the organism that holds the situation and history of the individual. It makes sense that miasm or miasmatic taint may be intimately connected with the ambient. This term is not used in the *Organon* but is included in the glossary to help define terms.

It is clear that Hahnemann treated diseases, that people could suffer from more than one disease at any one time, and that each disease is a dynamic whole, an entity, a creature or essence, with its own characteristic expression.

This suggests that each one requires its own individual medicinal treatment, and that one medicine is likely to be followed by another. In practice it often happens that a patient experiences a number of '*befallments*' or '*impinging potences*' within a very short time. A common example is a road traffic accident and its '*attendant circumstances*': shock and trauma, accompanied by blood loss and pain, complicated by anti-tetanus injection, analgesics, anaesthetics, surgery, more drugs, MRSA etc. Any of these events can, by themselves, mistune the life force. Taken together they may save the life **and** compromise the dynamis. Such a dynamic situation certainly calls for a dynamic practitioner, one who is aware of dynamics and able to participate in them; one who is able to prescribe one medicine after the other as appropriate to the needs of the life force.

Notes
○ Disease is a dynamic mistunement of the life force and therefore of the whole organism.
○ To fully cure the disease every aspect of it needs to be considered. This includes all changes in state, condition and appearance (as expressed through signs and symptoms), all possible aetiologies, relevant circumstances and traumas and any active miasmatic influences.

References
1. H.L. Chitkara. *Best of Burnett: James Compton Burnett.* B. Jain Publishers (P) Ltd., New Delhi, 1992, p. 66.

Symptoms

Dynamic mistunement, *'the suffering of the life force'* (Aph. 7) is expressed through signs and symptoms. These are changes in perception, behaviour, feeling, sensation and function. These changes may be experienced by the patient, noticed by his family and attendants or observed or sensed by the homoeopath.

The root of the word symptom is the Greek, syn-piptein, meaning 'to fall'. We 'fall ill' and we experience *'befallments'*. Maybe we fall out of unity into polarity, out of ease into dis-ease (see Psora). In 'falling ill', symptoms seem to fall out from the state of health and into an expression of the disease state (see Individualising Disease).

Symptoms form the vital language of the life force in the expression of its mistunement and its attempts to return to health.

Classification of Diseases

Hahnemann appears to suggest two ways of classifying diseases: according to their nature and according to their genesis or beginning.

Nature: either acute or chronic. An acute disease has a tendency to cease, to end in recovery or death, within a relatively short time. A chronic disease has a tendency to continue, to gradually and continuously mistune the life force over many years until the organism is destroyed.

Acute diseases may be further divided:

Individual acute diseases tend to be febrile and contained within a single person at any one time. A common example would be a 'flu-like' illness in someone who had been working too hard, or who had been frightened, chilled, or overheated. Hahnemann suggests that these types of disease are only passing flare-ups of an underling psoric condition that settles down again if the febrile state is not too severe.

Sporadic acute diseases affect a small number of people at the same time, in different locations. There is no obvious cause or connection.

Epidemic acute diseases induce very similar symptoms, with the same cause, in many people at the same time. These diseases tend to be highly contagious within areas where people are crowded together, such as slums, schools, hospitals, refugee camps, disaster areas and war zones. Some are well-known disease phenomena and are identified by a particular name such as cholera. Hahnemann called them '*acute miasms*' (see Miasm).

There are three kinds of **chronic diseases**:

Iatrogenic diseases are those caused by prolonged orthodox medical treatment. These are induced by drugs, surgery or other procedures and are responsible for thousands of hospital admissions, and deaths, every year. '*Of all the chronic diseases, these botchings of the human condition bought forth by the allopathic calamitous art (at its worst in recent times) are the saddest and most incurable.'* (Aph. 75) How much more so today?

The so-called '*pseudo-chronic*' diseases are those caused by environmental factors and lifestyle. These generally resolve themselves through simple changes in diet, habit and environment.

'*The true, natural, chronic diseases are those that arise from a chronic miasm.*' (Aph. 78) These diseases are considered more fully in the following chapters.

Genesis: this refers to how the disease begins.

Iatrogenic diseases are those caused by the doctor through actions or words. This now includes 'vaccinosis' (1).

Ideogenic diseases arise as a result of an impression made directly upon the mind by an external or internal influence. These include those that Hahnemann referred to as '*the highest' diseases, mistunements of the life principle brought about through the imagination* (Aph.17, fn.). A disturbing dream, image, or story might induce such a disease, as would something like a voodoo curse.

Ideogenic diseases also include emotional diseases '*which were first spun and maintained by the soul*' (Aph. 226). These progress '*outward from the emotional mind*' and are due to persistent and long-continued stresses such as fear, worry and abuse. In time these truly emotional diseases can destroy the physical health of the individual (Aph. 225). Hahnemann is clear that it is only these emotional diseases '*that allow themselves to be rapidly transformed into well-being of the soul by psychotherapeutic means*' (Aph. 226) and then only if the physical plane has not been too seriously affected. It makes sense to me also that it is these diseases that best suit the prescription of one medicine based upon its mental and emotional symptom similarity to the disease process. Even so, Hahnemann suggests that such diseases are based upon an undeveloped psoric miasm and that their treatment should end with an anti-psoric prescription.

Pathogenic diseases include those dynamic mistunements induced through infection by micro-organisms (miasms) or by poisons. These express themselves firstly through changes in sensation and function that are experienced generally or physically. Over time, the internal dynamic mistunement intensifies and the somatic expression begins to decrease as mental and emotional expression increases. A simple example of this might be 'despair, from itching of the skin' in psora. This can progress '*right up to the most striking one-sidedness until finally the disease transfers itself (almost like a local malady) to the invisibly subtle mental and emotional organs*' (Aph. 215, 216).

'*Almost all so-called mental and emotional diseases are nothing other than somatic diseases in which the symptom of mental and emotional mistunement that is peculiar to each disease heightens itself as the somatic symptoms diminish.*' (Aph. 215)

To Hahnemann's classification I find it useful to add *Traumagenic* diseases; disturbances in the life force caused by particular traumatic experiences. Traumas such as the death of a loved one, rape, physical injury, may have an ideogenic aspect yet it is the element of 'shock' that leads me to consider them as a distinct type of disease.

Also, we need to consider our increasing knowledge of genetics and epi-genetics and wonder about the possible connections with miasm.

References
1. James Compton Burnett. *Vaccinosis and Its Cure by Thuja.* B. Jain Publishers (P) Ltd., New Delhi, 1987.

Miasm

Hahnemann's theory of miasms seems to be the most contentious, debated and misunderstood aspect of homoeopathic medicine, particularly amongst homoeopaths! In essence we are looking at the effects of infectious diseases upon the human constitution.

How and why Hahnemann developed this theory is well documented in his *Chronic Diseases*. He noticed that while acute diseases responded well to homoeopathic treatment, chronic diseases seemed to continue and increase from year to year, despite robust constitutions, healthy living conditions and good diet. As far as the homoeopathic treatment of chronic diseases was concerned:

'Their beginning was promising, the continuation less favourable, the outcome hopeless.' (CD 5)

Hahnemann gathered together and studied many of his failed cases and so examined a huge totality of symptoms. After twelve years of investigation he came to the conclusion that the obstacle to cure in many cases seemed very often to be due to a former infectious disease process and its effects upon the life force organised as constitution. This was especially the case if such a process had been suppressed by *'faulty practice'*.

He discovered a symptom complex that seemed to underlie a whole range of apparently different diseases. Each symptom complex is the expression of one underlying dynamic mistunement in humanity, of which each individual expresses *'only a part'*. As described in aphorism 103, Hahnemann studied acute epidemic diseases as well as chronic diseases and found that each has its own individual dynamis, or energy pattern.

I am sure that Hahnemann would have chosen the Hippocratic word *'miasma/miasm'* carefully. It means: 'stain, pollution, defilement'. It is also interpreted as 'infective material', and in most dictionaries the word infect means 'to taint, pollute or contaminate'.

For Hahnemann miasma was not a concept, it was something real, a '*spirit-like*' potence, and an individual dynamis very capable of mistuning the human dynamis. In his *Lesser Writings* (page 758, in 1831!) he writes about the development of Asiatic cholera:

'*The most striking examples of infection and rapid spread of the cholera take place, as is well known, and as the public journals likewise inform us, in this way: on board ships in those confined spaces, filled with mouldy watery vapours, the cholera miasm finds a favourable element for its multiplication, and grows into an enormously increased brood of the excessively minute, invisible, living organisms so inimical to human life, of which the contagious matter of the cholera most probably consists.*'

Throughout his writings he uses terms such as '*miasmic animalcules*', '*germs*' (CD 56), '*disease-parasites*' (CD 40, fn). He also uses the terms '*infection*' and '*contagion*' to support his idea of the life force being 'dipped into' or 'spoiled' by an external impinging potence (G 297). Infection refers specifically to the dynamic and physical impingement by microbes whilst contagion is more suggestive of the purely dynamic aspect of an impingement, such as the effect of a disgusting sight upon the imagination (Aph. 11, fn).

This all equates with what is now known about microbial infection by external impinging potences known as bacteria, viruses, and parasites. Yet Hahnemann was not a materialist, he was a dynamist and understood that each microbe has a purely dynamic aspect, its own dynamis.

Of acute diseases he writes of '*these various, acute half-spiritual miasms…that - after they have penetrated the vital force*' (CD 39, fn.) induce their own characteristic disease process. This either kills the patient or he recovers. He also writes of psora as being a '*half-spiritual miasma*', which '*like a parasite seeks to inroot its hostile life in the human organism and to continue its life there*' (CD 165). '*Inrooting*', like '*impinging*', is dynamic and can only occur when the organism is susceptible.

It seems clear to me that Hahnemann was alive to the energy of microbes, to the potency of each miasma, to what is now known as 'virulence'. It follows that each individual miasma will induce a characteristic mistunement and symptom picture within an individual human, and within human being as a whole. This is similar to the process in a proving when a medicinal potence impinges upon the healthy human life force to induce its own characteristic mistunement and symptomatic expression.

In the various writings on miasm, and especially regarding psora, there seems to be confusion as to whether the term refers to the external impinging potence, the consequent disease, a 'pre-disposition', or even the original susceptibility (again, especially regarding psora). What follows represents my understanding based upon my most consistent reading of Hahnemann together with my observations in practice.

Miasma/miasm: The dynamic morbific potence, '*half spiritual*' and half physical, that impinges upon, dips into, spoils, or otherwise infects the human life force. These may induce acute or chronic diseases, according to their nature. As an example, acute epidemic diseases produce very similar symptoms in a large group of people who are experiencing similar circumstances, such as poverty and overcrowding. The circumstances create susceptibility in most people to the same external disease-inducing potence. This '*puts all those who have fallen ill into the same kind of disease process*' (Aph. 73).

'*Some acute epidemic diseases are particular acute miasms that recur in the same manner and are therefore known by a traditional name.*' (Aph. 73) Chickenpox, whooping cough, and cholera are examples. These are associated with a dynamic organism, observed and cultured, known as *Herpes zoster* (a virus), *Bordetella pertussis* and *Vibrio cholerae* (both bacteria) respectively.

An example of a chronic disease-causing miasma/miasm is *Treponema pallidum*. This spirochaete is the organically identifiable aspect of an external dynamic potence that induces a similar disease expression in a wide range of susceptible people. The disease is known as syphilis.

The miasma/miasm associated with a pathogenic disease may be 'passed on' to other people through different types of contact, or through the uterus, congenitally, as in syphilis or AIDS.

Miasmatic Disease: The miasma/miasm enters into intimate relationship with the human life force and disturbs or mistunes it. This is a miasmatic or infectious disease. It is an acquired disease in that person for one lifetime, and the process is the same for both acute and chronic diseases.

Firstly, *'the infection with miasmas takes place, without doubt, in one single moment'* (CD 37) at a time when the organism is most susceptible. The impingement is dynamically communicated to the whole of the life force *'in the same moment'* so that the dynamic mistunement is virtually instantaneous. Secondly, there is a period of time *'during which the entire organism is being penetrated by the disease'*. I understand this as being the time taken for the dynamic mistunement to become embodied. This is widely known as the incubation or prodromal period. Thirdly, the mistuned life force produces symptoms as an expression of its mistunement, and also as its best attempt to preserve the integrity of the organism. An acute disease will then run its course, often through a fever, a crisis and an eruption, and the organism will either recover or die.

In a chronic disease the primary symptom is external and local. In psora it is an itching, vesicular eruption; in syphilis a venereal chancre; in sycosis a venereal fig-wart. It is representative of the internal disease and acts as a safety valve for it, helping to *'alleviate and soothe'*, keeping it *'latent and confined'* (CD 45). At this stage the disease is *'most easily cured'* with appropriate homoeopathic treatment.

Without treatment the intensity of the internal disturbance or mistunement increases. Consequently, the external symptom also increases.

'While the presence of this local symptom silences the internal disease for a while, little is won on the side of the life force towards either diminishing the total malady or curing it. On the contrary, the internal suffering gradually increases and nature

is compelled to enlarge and worsen the local symptom more and more in order that it may still suffice as a representative for the enlarged internal disease and for its appeasement.' (Aph. 201)

Other than this local symptom, the patient may appear to be in good health. If, by external means, the local symptom, the safety valve or outlet, is denied or removed then suppression takes place and *'nature makes up for this by awaking the internal suffering'* and *'heightening the disease'* (Aph. 202). *'The sustentive power of life is therefore required to transfer the focus for the great internal malady to a still nobler site.'* (Aph. 205, fn.)

This means that a whole range of disease syndromes, characteristic of each underlying miasmatic disease *'must inevitably unfold and erupt, thus spreading all the nameless misery and the incredible quantity of chronic diseases which have tormented human kind for centuries and millennia'* (Aph. 204).

To be clear, *'the incredible quantity of chronic diseases'* and *'all the untold deficiencies, deteriorations, mistunements and sufferings'* (Aph. 81) represent the numerous manifestations of one underlying miasmatic disease mistunement. A disease which is *'unvarying'* in its dynamis. This is recognised in both the individual and the collective.

'These have been falsely listed in the pathology books under a multitude of names, as diseases existing in and of themselves.' (Aph. 81)

Between the suppression of the primary symptom and the proliferation of the secondary symptoms there is a latent period when the miasmatic mistunement is *'slumbering'*. Hahnemann suggests that the longer the external symptom is sustained before suppression, the swifter the production of secondary symptoms. Certainly, *'without the aid of art'* the latent miasmatic disease (especially psora) *'is ineradicable, and cannot be extirpated by the strength of even the best and most robust bodily constitution, and it will increase even to the end of the patient's life.'* (CD 49)

This internal disease can *'slumber'* for years and the person may appear to be well and healthy. *'However, it inevitably comes to the fore again in later years with adverse events and relationships in life.'* (Aph. 78, fn.) Such triggers can include grief, stress, life-style or suppressive treatments; anything that over-stimulates or undermines the constitution.

Once aroused, the chronic miasmatic disease process creates havoc and continues within the person for one lifetime.

It is important to bear in mind that whilst the progress of a chronic miasmatic disease appears to be inwards, from without, this is most definitely not the case. *'In these cases, one tends to say, incorrectly, that by external means the local malady has been driven back into the body or upon the nerves.'* (Aph. 202)

With continued suppression the internal mistunement is continually intensified or *'heightened'* and the increasingly compromised life force has to produce more and more inward symptoms in order to protect the centre yet also to alleviate the intensity of the disturbance. The *'mental and emotional organs'* of the Geist and the Gemüt are among the last to be directly affected in the progression of a chronic miasmatic disease. This is not to say that mental and emotional symptoms will not be produced but that they will arise out of somatic suffering. An example of this would be a suicidal depression arising out of intense physical pain. This is the opposite of the process in *'emotional diseases which are spun and maintained by the soul'*.

Hahnemann is clear: *'the maladies of the coarser bodily organs are, as it were, transferred and diverted onto the almost spiritual, mental and emotional organs, which have never been reached, and are unreachable, by any dissecting scalpel'* (Aph. 216, and, again, 215).

An acquired miasmatic disease can be dormant, latent, or active. Dormant means that there are no active symptoms of the disease but there is a record of it in the personal medical history. Latent means that there will be subtle symptoms of the disease, which will only be perceived by an attentive practitioner. In the active situation, the dynamic disease dominates the symptomatology.

An individual may suffer from one or more miasmatic diseases at any one time. Hahnemann asserts that by far the most frequent and fundamental chronic miasmatic disease is psora.

Miasmatic Taint or **Inheritance**: If a chronic miasmatic disease has mistuned the life force/constitution of a parent, that mistunement may affect the dynamis of any offspring at the moment of conception. It may be present energetically in the offspring as a dis-rhythm, groove, rut, fault, trait, stain, seed, wound, echo or shadow within the life force. Essentially this represents the effects of the ancestral disease upon the individual. No miasm is present, only the energetic ripples of its mistunement. What is present is a miasmatic attunement. This expresses itself as a tendency, a susceptibility and a pre-disposition to disease. The more intense and long-lasting the disease in the ancestor the greater the possible tendency within the offspring. This potential for disease may be activated at any time in the life of the individual by triggers such as grief, poor nutrition etc.

A miasmatic inherited taint may be dormant or active and is often identified through the family medical history. A common example from practice is a tendency to upper respiratory tract infections in a child with a tubercular ancestor. Whilst any individual may possess a number of taints, generally one will predominate at any one time.

Miasmatic Quality: This refers to a quality of being, of being diseased, or of behaving, which is natural to the individual (or his family) and which resonates with the quality of a given miasmatic influence yet which does not stem from a known miasmatic infection in the ancestral past. An example of this could be destructiveness. Destructiveness is a quality that we homoeopaths refer to as being 'syphilitic', yet it does not necessarily mean that the disease of syphilis has occurred within the family. Some homoeopathic observers have suggested that such qualities in the human being have come solely from the miasmatic influences; that destructiveness, as an example, has arisen upon the Earth as a result of people having syphilis. It makes more sense to me that the quality of destructiveness would have arisen spontaneously and naturally as part of having to 'kill or be killed'. Perhaps people who particularly either enjoyed or suffered from this aspect of life would be more susceptible to a potence such as *Treponema*. It makes sense that the quality of destructiveness could have been intensified by the disease process within many people over time, but not caused by it.

Miasmatic Nosode: This is a medicine prepared from the end results of a miasmatic disease. An example would be the sputum taken from a person suffering with tuberculosis. Such a medicine can be extremely useful in the treatment of an active miasmatic disease or in the lessening of a miasmatic tendency. It appears to have little influence in the lessening of a miasmatic quality.

Hahnemann's use of the term '*anti-miasmatic*' may suggest a resonance with the allopathic prescription of an anti-biotic. This is not the case. A chronic miasma '*can only be exterminated and annihilated by a counter infection, by means of the potency of a medicinal disease quite similar to it and stronger than it…*' (CD 40, fn.)

The observation that the fundamental cause of a chronic disease mostly rests upon the effects of a preceding infectious disease, especially one that has been suppressed, either in an individual or an ancestor, makes a lot of sense. Consider the degree of suffering caused to humanity by leprosy, sepsis, syphilis etc. and the number of people killed by tuberculosis, smallpox, malaria and now AIDS. Over millennia and through hundreds of generations these miasmatic diseases have ravaged the human constitution. The miasmatic inheritance is the effect and current expression of that ravaging. The human life force has been mistuned to an increasing susceptibility to disease and the evidence is all around us.

In my own practice I have seen the after-effects of diseases such as influenza, glandular fever, pneumonia, tuberculosis, hepatitis, and observed how long it can take for people to restore their constitution, their healthiest state.

It seems to me that Hahnemann's work on chronic disease is incomplete yet it represents an astonishing beginning. *The Chronic Diseases* remains amongst the earliest pieces of epidemiological research known.

Since Hahnemann we have learnt of the great value of improved living and working conditions, better sanitation and public health measures. These have helped to greatly reduce the incidence of infectious disease… yet tuberculosis is returning to our communities, MRSA is rampant in our hospitals. As homoeopaths we need to be ready, now.

Resources

1. R.E. Dudgeon. *The Lesser Writings of Samuel Hahnemann*. B. Jain Publishers (P) Ltd., 2001
2. James Tyler Kent. *Lectures on Homoeopathic Philosophy*. B. Jain Publishers (P) Ltd., New Delhi, 1987, chapters 18 and 19.
3. Processo Sanchez Ortega. *Notes on the Miasms*. National Homoeopathic Pharmacy, New Delhi, 1980.
4. Subrata Kumar Banerjea. *Miasmatic Prescribing*. Allen College of Homoeopathy, Essex, England, 2001.
5. George Dimitriadis. *The Theory of Chronic Diseases According to Hahnemann*. Hahnemann Institute of Homoeopathy, Sydney, 1992.

Miasm Essentials

- Miasm: an external potence, '*half spiritual*' and half physical, capable of inducing a characteristic disease mistunement in the life force of a living organism.

- Miasmatic infection: the process through which the miasmatic potence impinges upon, dips into or spoils, the life force of the susceptible individual. Both internal susceptibility and external potence are necessary. It is not a question of either/or; it is a matter of and/both.

- Miasmatic disease: a mistunement due to that impinging potence. This can be acute or chronic.

- Miasmatic taint: an attunement to disease that is characteristic of the miasm.

- Miasmatic attunement: a set of susceptibilities, either acquired or inherited, resulting from a miasmatic disease in self or ancestor.

- Miasmatic nosode: a specific re-tuning potence made from the primary lesion of the miasmatic disease.

Psora

'Psora is that most ancient, most universal, most destructive, and yet most misapprehended chronic miasmatic disease which for many thousands of years has disfigured and tortured mankind.' (CD 11)

The word itself is confusing. In Hahnemann's time it was used to describe a whole variety of skin affections such as leprosy, St. Anthony's fire (a spreading streptococcal infection of the skin), herpes and tinea. Deriving from the Greek word for 'itch', psora was also used in the narrow sense for scabies, a skin infestation associated with the 'itch mite' *Sarcoptes scabiei*. Most authors writing on psora focus on scabies despite the fact that Hahnemann does not even mention it in either the *Organon* or *Chronic Diseases*. He was, of course, aware of it but probably saw it as more of an aggravating or predisposing factor (1).

Roberts (2) writes that the word comes from an original Hebrew word, Tsorat, meaning: 'a groove, a fault, a pollution, a stigma; often applied to leprous manifestations and the Great Plague'. Certainly within *The Chronic Diseases* Hahnemann writes about an *'occidental'* leprosy, its moderation over time and its eventual suppression.

Within the Bible the Hebrew word Tzaraat, or Tsara'ath, was used to describe a state of impurity associated with several skin diseases, possibly including 'leprous manifestations' but not the leprosy known today as Hansen's disease.

We may conclude that psora includes a wide range of impinging potences, such as bacteria, viruses, fungi and mites, which induce a wide range of skin eruptions.

'As long as humanity has existed, people have been exposed, individually or collectively, to illnesses from physical or moral causes. In the raw state of nature few means of aid were needed, since the simple way of life admitted but few diseases. With civilisation, however, the occasions for falling ill, and the need for help against diseases grew in equal measure.' (Intro. p. 8)

This suggests that Hahnemann considered the susceptibility to disease to have always been an aspect of human being. It also suggests that life became more complex as humans became more civilised. This was mirrored in more complex disease processes and the subsequent increase in complex, and potentially suppressive, treatments.

It makes sense to me that the most fundamental aspect of human being is the struggle to stay alive, to survive on the surface of this planet. To survive we have to meet certain needs within us, we have to find those life essentials that we lack. By this I mean that we all need clean food and water, shelter and warmth, safety. Then we need community and, with this, law and morality. As we gather together, life becomes more complex and sanitation, food provision etc. become issues again.

This life is uncertain and involves struggle, success and failure, loss, grief, sorrow and an anxiety that is always somewhere around. This struggle renders us susceptible to disease potencies, to dynamic infection. Acute diseases and those associated with psora (and pseudo-psora, or tuberculosis - see later) are those most associated with poverty, with poor living and working conditions and the mental and emotional stresses involved in surviving such situations. These basic situations can be seen in so-called 'third world' countries, or in the aftermath of wars, hurricanes or earthquakes. Increasingly we see them in so-called 'developed countries' too, with mass unemployment, junk food, inner-city breakdown and the consequent sense of stress, failure and futility. It seems reasonable to suggest that 'scratching a living' is the most basic cause of mistunement in both the collective and the individual human life force.

Kent writes of the 'spiritual sickness', the thinking and willing of wrongs that gave rise to the susceptibility to psora (3). This equates with the idea of 'the fall of man' and the Biblical story of Adam and Eve, of the concept of original sin and the 'fruit of the tree of the knowledge of good and evil'. Kent states that psora laid the foundation for other diseases:

'First there was the thinking of falses and willing of evils, thinking such falses as led to depraved living and a longing for what was not one's own, until finally action prevailed. The miasms which succeeded psora were but the outward representations of actions, which have grown out of thinking and willing.' (4)

Whilst there is much in Kent's thinking, Hahnemann did **not** suggest that psora gave rise to **all** disease. '*Psora... has become the mother of all the thousands of incredibly various (acute and) chronic (**non-venereal**) diseases, by which the whole civilized human race on the inhabited globe is being more and more afflicted.*' (CD 11; my emphasis.)

Other writers have taken Kent's view further by suggesting that psora arose at that point in human evolution where Life became conscious of itself. Julian Carlyon writes: '...the vast original malady is nothing less than the world-shattering effects of the emergence of human self-consciousness on the evolutionary scene.' (5)

Mythologically, the development of self-consciousness is described as a wound in the fabric of Life on Earth, a sundering of the unconscious wholeness. It seems reasonable to suppose that self-consciousness would come with a sense of separation, of alone-ness. This is likely to separate us from ease, make us un-easy, susceptible. This dis-ease might manifest as anxiety, with a sense of something missing, of inadequacy or inferiority, perhaps.

Maybe psora, as the original susceptibility to disease, is simply the result of the sudden perception in humans of polarity: 'I am: you are: I am separate: I am alone.' An understanding of polarity enables us to perceive that 'I am alone' is a delusion, a misperception. The reality is more likely to be, 'we are one'. The emotional response to 'I am alone' could be 'and I am afraid', and it is easy to see how such an anxiety could induce tension, mistunement, or dis-rhythm within the life force.

With polarity comes choice: 'the knowledge of good and evil'. We can choose evil, choose to go against our instinctive nature, 'to transgress' (6) or to sin. This may also induce tension, mistunement, dis-rhythm within the life force.

So, maybe the original susceptibility to disease has arisen because of an awareness of polarity, of living in a polarised world. Maybe it is simply a direct consequence of polarity. Maybe the universe is unfolding just as it should be. Maybe the cosmic dance continues until every possibility between mother tincture and infinity has been experienced. If the Great Mystery (Unity, Singularity) is experiencing itself through seemingly endless cycles of life and death then 'the fall', 'evil', sickness, simply have to be experienced as much as 'redemption', 'good', health, if wholeness or unity is to be re-experienced. Maybe 'to err is human' and it's OK. Maybe it is not a question of 'either/or', maybe it is 'and/both'.
Maybe not.
What do you think?

I am suggesting that the original susceptibility to most disease potences (other than those which induce acute or venereal diseases) may have arisen, and be continuing to arise, in one or more of the following ways:

- As a result of the stresses of surviving on planet Earth:
  'How on Earth will I survive?' 'I must struggle to adapt.'

- As a result of 'evil thinking':
  'Oh God I have sinned.' 'I must atone through the sweat of my brow.'

- As a result of self-consciousness:
  'I am: I am separate: I am alone.' 'I must think.'

- As a direct consequence of living in a polarised universe:
  'I am incomplete: I lack: I am poor.' 'I must work, to fulfil or enrich myself.'

Each of these possibilities suggests struggle and all could easily give rise to a state of anxiety. Anxiety can be described as an intense state of dis-ease or nervousness. This particular state of anxiety could be described as 'existential'.

It seems to me that anxiety can be expressed as a 'hyper' state; of sensitivity, activity, irritability and nervous restlessness. It can also be expressed as a 'hypo' state; of timidity, inhibition and lack of reaction. It also makes sense that both states will be expressed somatically. The commonly described view that psora is purely to do with hypofunction has never really made total sense to me.

It is also commonly written that psora produces almost no structural change but largely functional disorders. When Hahnemann describes the '*countless forms of disease*' which psora can produce he writes of '*hysteria, mania, epilepsy, scrofula, bone caries, cancer, neoplasms, kidney stones*' and many more (Aph. 80). These are all high-energy, tissue-proliferating and destructive disease processes! What makes most sense to me is that psora encompasses all manner of dysfunction, including the hyper and perverted functions of the venereal diseases, yet with its own characteristic expression of them.

As well as '*most ancient*' and '*most destructive*', Hahnemann describes psora as the '*most universal*' miasm. This seems to be because almost all people are susceptible to it at some time. Also, psora is extremely infectious by nature. '*No other chronic miasma infects more generally, more surely, more easily and more absolutely than the miasma of itch.*' (CD 42)

Hahnemann is clear that psora is only infectious at the stage of the primary symptoms. Only the fluid-filled vesicles of the itching eruption '*contain the communicable miasma of the Psora*'. Secondary symptoms '*cannot at all communicate this disease to others*' (CD 45).

Hahnemann does not write that all other miasms arise from psora. Neither does he write that every body is psoric. He writes that, despite suffering many acute epidemic diseases, he himself had '*never been afflicted with the Psora*' (CD 50, fn).

Psora is far too huge a study to cover adequately here. I encourage us all to continue reading Hahnemann, especially in *The Chronic Diseases*, until psora is more clearly understood.

References

1. Francisco Xavier Eizayaga. *Treatise on Homoeopathic Medicine.* Edicione Marcel, Buenos Aires, 1991, p. 289.
2. Herbert A. Roberts. *The Principles and Art of Cure by Homoeopathy.* B. Jain Publishers (P) Ltd., New Delhi, 1985, p. 184.
3. James Tyler Kent. *Lectures on Homoeopathic Philosophy.* B. Jain Publishers (P) Ltd., New Delhi, 1987, p.146.
4. James Tyler Kent. *Lectures on Homoeopathic Philosophy.* B. Jain Publishers (P) Ltd., New Delhi, 1987, p.157.
5. Julian Carlyon. *Understanding Homoeopathy, Homoeopathic Understanding.* Helios Homoeopathy Ltd., Kent, England, 2003, p.136.
6. Processo Sanchez Ortega. *Notes on the Miasms.* National Homoeopathic Pharmacy, New Delhi, 1980, p. 66.

The Essential Characteristics of Chronic Miasmatic Diseases and Inheritances

This study is much bigger than is allowed for here. What follows are the most basic yet confirming features verified through practice. The characteristics that are the clearest, most viable and most reflective of the miasmatic disease process tend to be general and physical in nature, rather than mental or emotional. Again, what follows is minimal. This material needs a book all to itself.

Psora

Psora represents a mistunement of the life force in the sense of lack, of deficiency. A lack of nutrients, or of the ability to assimilate them, leads to a persistent hunger. The lack of energy or stamina leads to fatigue and the particular hunger for sweet food. Lack of warmth or vital heat means that the patient is generally chilly, while the dryness (skin, stool, cough, hair) that pervades this miasmatic influence arises from a lack of moisture. A lack of reaction is expressed through relapsing states, slow recovery from acute illnesses and the inability to respond to a well-indicated medicine.

As if to try and compensate for this lack, there is a constant desire for stimulation on all levels. Psora also manifests a hyper-reactivity as evidenced by extreme sensitivity (allergy etc.) on all levels.

Psora has a particular affinity for the skin inducing all kinds of eruptions that are characterized by a profound itching. Itching, burning and redness run throughout the body.

The psoric mistunement is aggravated by:
Suppressions, of all kinds
Emotions, most especially long-lasting grief and sorrow

Wind and cold air
Full moon, menstrual cycles, seasons (i.e. periodically)

And ameliorated by:
Warmth
Eating good food
Discharges, especially perspiration and diarrhoea

We observe:
Periodic sick headaches
Cradle cap, dandruff: dry, scabby and itchy
Premature white hair

Daylight photophobia
Muscae volitantes

Irritability from smell; with nausea
Irritability from noise

Unwashed looking face
Red lips, as if on fire

Burnt taste in the mouth

Empty, all-gone, hollow feeling in abdomen; always hungry, at night, for sweet food
Parasitic worms

Lots of sexual thoughts but inhibited action; masturbation

Cramps in calves and feet
Burning in palms and soles
Coldness in hands and feet

Psychological characteristics mainly relate to the existential struggle to survive. Great mental activity goes on around an inferiority complex and lack of confidence. Existential anxiety can manifest in specific fears such as fear of dark, death, night, being alone, poverty, robbers, misfortune, failure and disease. There is a profound despair, of survival or recovery, and from itching of the skin. This last symptom is an extreme expression of the purely psoric suffering.

The dynamic of psora is one of struggle and the statement seems to be: 'I am alone and I am afraid, and it's hard work staying alive!'

There is often a past personal or family medical history of: Skin 'diseases' and allergies; the classic 'atopic terrain'.

Predominantly 'anti-psoric' medicines (medicines that produce similar dynamic infections) include: Baryta carbonica, Calcarea carbonica, Lycopodium, Sulphur, Graphites, Kali carbonicum, Petroleum, Natrum muriaticum and Psorinum.

Pseudo-psora or Tuberculosis

Hahnemann originally listed tubercular phenomena under psora (e.g. scrofula, laryngeal pthisis, consumption, pulmonary consumption (CD 93), but the rise of tuberculosis suggested itself as a miasm in its own right. Its organic aspect is recognised as *Mycobacterium tuberculosis* and it induces its own characteristic disease process. It is easy to identify psoric, syphilitic and even sycotic tones within tuberculosis yet it is not a mixture; it has its own unique dynamis.

Tuberculosis is a mistunement in the sense of constriction, of suffocation. This is expressed primarily through the respiratory system via syndromes such as pneumonia, emphysema, haemoptysis, croup, whooping cough and asthma. There is a sensation of constriction, of suffocation, of tightness, that is worsened by a close atmosphere and helped by open air, especially mountain air. This miasm induces a chronic and recurring inflammation of the glands, such as tonsils and adenoids (especially in children), accompanied by a sensation of constriction or closing in.

There is an intense restlessness of the mind and body, and a great susceptibility to change. Changes in the weather can affect the tubercular individual profoundly and symptoms are always changing – in degree and location. There is a strong desire for change as well as a distinct amelioration from it.

The tubercular individual is highly energetic yet burns up or consumes this energy and so often presents with great fatigue and a feeling of always being tired. Always tired and always hungry too, with an appetite described as 'ravenous', he never gains weight and is more likely to lose it.

There is a great sensitivity on all levels of the organism: sensitivity to acute miasms and upper respiratory tract infections ('catches cold easily') with a tendency to complications in childhood acute diseases and relapsing and recurring states. Allergy and hay fever are common examples of this sensitivity, and hyper-kinesis is an example of this combined with the restlessness and energy of the tubercular child.

The tubercular mistunement is generally aggravated by:
Constriction of any sort, such as a close atmosphere, a marriage, a mortgage or a baby car seat!
Physical exertion, especially when so fatigued
Seasons, menstrual cycles, phases in life such as adolescence or the middle passage

And is ameliorated by:
Being in the mountains
Cool open air and wind upon the face
Nosebleeds, especially in children
Change

We observe:
Epilepsy
Periodic sick headaches, weekend migraines and menstrual headaches

Astigmatism
Chronic dilatation of the pupil
Teenage acne
Blue rings around the eyes
Chronic, recurring tonsillitis
Perforated ear drum, after otitis
Chronic, recurring nosebleeds

Easy decay of teeth, early in life
Salty, bloody taste

Desire for stimulating food; salt, smoked meats and fish
Desire for milk, ice cream

Persistent bedwetting

Very sexual
Periods painful, profuse, too early, long lasting

Poor chest development, lack of space means lack of air which gives rise
to a sensation of constriction and shortness of breath.

Cold, clammy hands and feet
Brittle nails
Softening of bones, osteoporosis

Profuse perspiration, at night or on exertion.

Psychological characteristics relate to an intensification of day-to-day
survival issues with a profound feeling of constriction and dissatisfaction.
This gives rise to restlessness and a desire for change and travel, to
changing moods and contradictory behaviour. Everything is expressed
with characteristic intensity.

The dynamic of tuberculosis is one of extreme restlessness and the
statement seems to be: 'I must go!'

There is often a past personal or family medical history of:
Tuberculosis and respiratory 'diseases' of all kinds
Glandular Fever
Recurrent tonsillitis, or tonsils and adenoids removed
Allergies
Ringworm

Predominantly 'anti-tubercular' medicines include: Calcarea phosphorica, Drosera, Iodum, Phosphorus, Silica, Stannum and Tuberculinum.

Syphilis

The organic aspect of this miasmatic influence has been identified as the spirochaete organism *Treponema pallidum*. This '*half-spiritual*' miasma induces a dynamic mistunement in the sense of perversion. This means 'to go the wrong way' and leads to a constriction of Life's abundance, to destruction, decay and early death.

There is a profound destruction of tissues through processes such as ulceration, caries and necrosis. Discharges from such processes are often offensive or bloody. There is much physical deformity and stunted growth.

Syphilis has an affinity for the bones, especially the long bones, and symptoms are often described as 'violent', for example 'dreadful pains' and corrosive discharges.

The syphilitic mistunement is generally aggravated:
At night
During the cold of winter and the heat of summer
By drinking alcohol

And is ameliorated:
During the day
In the mountains
When ulcers appear on the skin

We observe:
'Skeletal' head and facial features
'T-shaped' headaches
Total alopecia
Keratitis, worse 2-5 a.m.
Caries of mastoid
'Saddle nose' as nasal bones are destroyed by caries
Caries and crumbling of teeth
Hutchinson's teeth, cleft palate, hare lip
Metallic taste in mouth
Jaw over- or under-shot
Ulceration in throat
Perverted appetite; often an aversion to food, or a desire for cold food and alcohol
Obstinate constipation

Swollen and indurated testicles
Sterility
Tendency to abort; multiple abortions
Cervical and labial ulceration

Arrhythmia: with palpitations, at night
Aortic aneurysm

Severe pain in the long bones
Insomnia, from tormenting ideas
Gangrene
Varicose ulcers, with a putrid discharge

Profuse, offensive, sticky and excoriating perspiration, which does not relieve

Psychological characteristics relate to a destruction of the sense of self worth; the value of Life itself has been eroded. This is expressed through a loathing of life, rancour, profound depression, suicide and genocide.

Full of fears: death, dying, darkness, losing control, insanity, AIDS, contamination. There can also be a profound obsessional neurosis.

The dynamic of syphilis is one of perversion and the statement seems to be: 'I will kill or be killed'.

There is often a past personal or family medical history of:
Many immature deaths
Very few offspring
Insanity
Suicide
Tuberculosis
Alcoholism
Syphilis

Predominantly 'anti-syphilitic' medicines include: Arnica, Arsenicum iodatum, Aurum metallicum, Aurum muriaticum natronatum, Kali iodatum, Mercurius, Phytolacca, Syphilinum and Uranium nitricum.

Sycosis

This 'fig wart miasma' does not seem to have a currently identifiable organic aspect. *Neisseria gonorrhoeae* is the microbe most often associated with '*the other, common gonorrhoea*' (CD 99) but is not known to produce 'fig warts'. This may, in part, explain why Thuja is a more effective 'anti-sycotic' medicine than the nosode Medorrhinum.

Sycosis represents a mistunement in the sense of expansion, over-growth and excess. It produces growths, tumours, warts and polyps in the fibrous and soft tissues of the body. 'Gonorrhoea is the mother of all catarrh' said Burnett, and excess catarrh, and pus, is found in the mucous membranes and pelvic cavity. This type of catarrhal discharge often has a fishy smell and is characteristically yellow-green in colour. Catarrh and pus seem to somehow crystallize out in the process of grit (in joints especially) and stone formation. The ill-effects of vaccination (known as 'vaccinosis') are also resonant with the expression of this sycosis.

The sycotic mistunement is generally aggravated:
During the day
By cold, damp weather

And is ameliorated:
By discharges
As warts appear
By warmth

We observe:
Ophthalmia neonatoram; profuse, purulent, green/yellow discharge
Excess hair; face, arms, legs, back
Fishy taste in the mouth
Desire for too much food
Craving for flesh

Diarrhoea is an outstanding feature; profuse and explosive
Sensation of animals moving in the abdomen

Urethritis, cystitis
Prostatic enlargement

Gonorrhoea
Genital warts
Cysts, fibroids
Endometriosis, ovaritis, Bartholin's abscess
Severe menstrual colic
Fishy discharges, offensive moistness of genitals

Humid asthma
Sudden heart attacks
Arthritis, worse for cold and damp
Nails are thick and ridged

Warts, moles, spider naevi
Oily, greasy skin
Herpes zoster - chickenpox/shingles

The psychological characteristics relate to having an abundance of desires and the hurried need to get them met. Greed, lust and ambition give rise to a secretiveness and mistrust. There is often a deep sense of shame or guilt to which the person responds by trying to cover up, hide or escape. This can give rise to paranoia about being found out and an increasing rigidity in behaviour.

The dynamic of sycosis is one of expansion and the statement seems to be: 'I want it all and I want it now, but I don't want to be seen as this'.

There is often a previous personal or family medical history of:
Warts
Pelvic or genital infections, inflammations or growths

Predominantly 'anti-sycotic' medicines include: Argentum nitricum, Medorrhinum, Natrum sulphuricum and Thuja.

Cancer

Cancer may not be a truly Hahnemannian miasmatic disease because there is no known external potence which induces it (except in specific cancers such as Burkitt's lymphoma). It may, however, have developed from the continuing and increasing suppression of all the other acute and chronic miasmatic processes over time. This would also include the suppression of acute inflammatory processes in childhood through immunisation, antibiotics and steroids. What is certain is that the field of cancer is clearly recognised as both a chronic disease process and an inherited predisposition.

Cancer is a mistunement in the sense of suppression, repression and oppression. This tends to general de-pression of the sense of self. Inflammatory conditions are suppressed and tumoral conditions arise, including many kinds of cancer. The field of cancer may be supported, and health undermined, by increasing pollution both of the individual and his environment. Increasing sensitivity to the environment has become a feature as expressed through allergies to such substances as petroleum-based products, food additives, peanuts and even bread. Symptoms are often contradictory and include those of the other miasmatic modulations.

The cancer mistunement is generally aggravated:
When alone
While thinking of his ailments
And ameliorated:
In company
When occupied

We observe:
Café au lait complexion
Facial tics and grimaces
Bluish sclerotics
Cracks at the corner of the mouth
Causeless, long-continued insomnia
Allergies of all kinds

Psychological characteristics relate to the sense of self having been undermined, squashed, crushed, dominated or denied. A healthy emotional life has not been allowed, and even healthy disease processes have been denied expression. Factors contributing to this mistunement might include two World Wars, mass vaccinations, antibiotics, steroids, birth control drugs, mass production of foodstuffs and stifling cultural norms. There is a profound sense of duty, too much responsibility at a young age, a pressure to conform and a pathological need to please others. Fear of not pleasing, of getting it wrong, can lead to an over-industriousness and fastidiousness. Other fears include: cancer, losing control of one's self, failure and a general background fear that is difficult to name.

The dynamic of cancer is to deny, and the statement seems to be: 'I am fine!' when it is clear that all is not well.

There is often a past personal medical history of a lot of childhood illnesses, all treated suppressively, or of no childhood illnesses at all, and glandular fever. There may be a family medical history that includes almost any kind of serious degenerative disease such as cancer, T.B., lupus, pernicious anaemia, rheumatoid arthritis and schizophrenia.

Predominantly 'anti-cancer' medicines include: Carcinosin, Conium, Lac caninum, Lac humanum, Lachesis, Nux vomica, Natrum muriaticum and Staphysagria.

Other potentially chronic miasmatic disease potences need to be researched and elucidated. These might include malaria, leprosy, polio and A.I.D.S. There is a lot of work to be done!

It is important to acknowledge the recent work of Rajan Sankaran in this area of study. It is also important to be clear that, however useful this work is, Sankaran's miasms are not the same as Hahnemann's.

Sources

1. Samuel Hahnemann. *The Chronic Diseases - Their Peculiar Nature and Their Homoeopathic Cure* (Theoretical Part, completed in 1838). B. Jain Publishers (P) Ltd., New Delhi, 1996 and 2005.
2. Processo Sanchez Ortega. *Notes on the Miasms.* National Homoeopathic Pharmacy, New Delhi, 1980.
3. Phyllis Speight. *A Comparison of the Chronic Miasms.* Health Science Press, 1977.
4. Subrata Kumar Banerjea. *Miasmatic Prescribing.* Allen College of Homoeopathy, Essex, England, 2001.
5. Harimohon Choudhury. *Indications of Miasms.* B. Jain Publishers (P) Ltd., New Delhi, 1988.
6. Personal notes from classes given by Sheilagh Creasey at the College of Classical Homoeopathy, Devon, 1988-9.
7. Clinical experiences and conversations with Ken Metson between 1991 and 1996.

Resources

1. Misha Norland with Claire Robinson. *Signatures: Miasms: AIDS - Spiritual Aspects of Homeopathy.* Yondercott Press, Abergavenny, U.K., 2003.

2. Ian Watson. *Understanding The Miasms: A Seminar With Ian Watson* (Recorded live in Sutton Coldfield, 27th October, 1996). Ian Watson Seminars Incorporating Cutting Edge Publications, 2004.

3. Rajan Sankaran. *The Substance of Homoeopathy.* Homoeopathic Medical Publishers, Mumbai, India, 1999.

4. Rajan Sankaran. *An Insight into Plants, Volume 1.* Homoeopathic Medical Publishers, Mumbai, India, 2002.

5. Peter Fraser. *The AIDS Miasm.* Biddles, Guildford, England, 2002.

Individualising Disease

Central to any consideration of homoeopathic medicine is the observation that every human being, every patient, is unique and that his disease state will, in some way, be an expression of that uniqueness, an expression of his individuality.

For the homoeopath the most important symptoms are those that most clearly express the individual nature of the patient and his disease. Grouped together these symptoms represent *'the outwardly reflected image of the inner wesen of the disease'* (Aph. 7).

Hahnemann's *'symptom complex'* refers to the fewest symptoms that most characterise the individual way in which the patient both creates and expresses his disease. The symptoms that have the greatest value are those that are the most *'striking, exceptional, unusual and odd (characteristic)'* (Aph. 153); those that are strange, rare and peculiar. Symptoms that are most useful in individualising a case of disease are those that are also clear, intense and spontaneously expressed to the homoeopath.

When the image of a natural disease (symptom complex) is matched with the image of a very similar proving disease (medicine picture) *'the disease is lifted and extinguished without significant ailment'* (Aph. 155).

This matching is a great part of the art of homoeopathy.

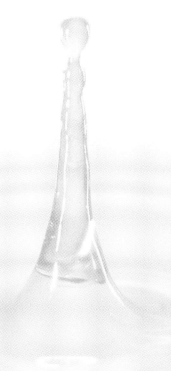

4

Part Four : The Homoeopath

The Unprejudiced Observer

'The unprejudiced observer, even the most sharp witted one - knowing the nullity of supersensible speculations which are not born out in experience - perceives nothing in each single case of disease other than the alterations in the condition of the body and soul, disease signs, befallments, symptoms, which are outwardly discernible through the senses. That is, the unprejudiced observer only perceives the deviations from the former healthy state of the now sick patient, which are:
1. felt by the patient himself,
2. perceived by those around him, and
3. observed by the physician.
All these perceptible signs represent the disease in its entire extent, that is, together they form the true and only conceivable gestalt of the disease.' (Aph. 6)

We now know that it is impossible to be an unprejudiced observer. The world does not happen out there, apart from us: we participate in its happening. The observer is part of the observation; the experimenter is part of the experiment. To every attempt at objectivity I cannot help but bring my subjective self.

What to do?

To be fully present, to be as focussed as possible in the here and now, seems to be the only way to avoid pre-judging. In this way the person and I are collaborative explorers and neither of us know quite what it is that we will find. Keeping open to all possibilities allows for a more thorough exploration. This involves fluidity and a kind of innocence.

> 'Attending fully and becoming supple,
> Can you be as a newborn babe?'
>
> *Lao Tsu*

Impossible as it may be to achieve, it seems to me that the spirit of Hahnemann's *'unprejudiced observer'* is telling us to get ourselves as much out of the way as we can and to focus upon the patient: only in this way can the patient and his disease be individualised. Acknowledging our own prejudices and working to minimise their impact upon our therapeutic relationships is a big part of homoeopathic practice. The discipline involved in this work sustains our integrity as true natural scientists.

Sound observation, using all our *'healthy senses'*, is important. Keeping our senses healthy is equally so.

Aware Participation

I am a unique and individual dynamic as much as the patient is. When we sit down together, life force to life force, we create a field around us, one that is individual to us. It is my task to sustain the clarity and integrity of that potentially therapeutic space or container so that the patient may enter into a dynamic relationship with myself and, through this, into a more intimate relationship with himself. This therapeutic relationship is established when the quality of my attention and intention is such that the person I am working with feels enough trust between us to be able to express himself freely.

Simply by being present in the field of the consultation I participate through my life force, organised in its different ways. The more fully I am present the greater is my conscious awareness of what is happening in the field, the greater the clarity of the information exchanged, and the greater the potency of the consultation, the relationship and the prescription. Gaining and sustaining this awareness is a life of work and practice, allowing me to know myself more and more.

I am the instrument through which all the information arising during the consultation is experienced, registered, analysed and prescribed upon. My task is to maintain and sustain the dynamic clarity and tone of this 'living healthy instrument'.

The Dynamic Practitioner

To be a dynamic practitioner one needs to practice dynamically. This means to work with energy. Firstly, it means to work with the energy of oneself, to be aware of it, to know its nature, its quality, how it is moving. The dynamic practitioner is the instrument upon which the patient makes a dynamic impression. For this to happen the practitioner has to allow the patient dynamis to enter into his field, and must be mindful of everything which happens there as a result. For this to be safe, the practitioner needs to be aware of his own dynamis and what is happening inside himself.

Secondly, it means to work with the energy of the patient. This means to be with it, to enter into relationship with it, to experience it, to move with it. This involves holistic participation. To work with the patient is to enter into the life and the disease, to enter into the streaming life force just long enough and deeply enough to receive enough of an impression to make a dynamic prescription. Again, for this to be safe the practitioner needs to know what is his energy and what is not, and to take care that this does not contaminate the patient's field. In this therapeutic relationship both people will be touched in some way.

Thirdly, it means to work with the energy of the medicine, to enter into dynamic relationship with the medicine (through provings and treatment) and to be aware of the curative process that it induces through its relationship with a susceptible human being.

The dynamic practitioner works in the here and now, with things as they are. He works with clarity and simplicity.

Restoration of Health

'The physician's highest and only calling is to make the sick healthy, to cure, as it is called.' (Aph. 1)

This is the work of the dynamic practitioner: the restoration of the former healthiest state of his patient. To restore means 'to make whole again', to reconnect him to his deeper self and enable him to live his life fully and with authenticity. Attending to him and prescribing medicines and offering sound advice over time can achieve this aim.

Healing and recovery happen of themselves, the wisdom of the body-mind an everyday miracle. Cure is always the result of art, of medicine.

'The highest ideal of cure is the rapid, gentle and permanent restoration of health.' (Aph. 2)

This mission statement is clear, and no sane practitioner of medicine will argue against it. It is not always achievable, yet it is that to which we can all aspire. Being involved in the process of cure, of participating in the restoration of even one person's health, is an up-lifting and restorative experience for both patient and practitioner. It is also very humbling.

'Any profession, no matter how humble, offers the possibility of satisfying a quest for the meaning of life, as long as it is practised with integrity. Thus the dignity of the task depends on who carries it out and how it is carried out, rather than what is actually done. Precisely because humility is required, the art of medicine is an occupation of the highest spiritual order.' (1)

Privilege comes to mind.

References

1. T.P. Paschero. *Homoeopathy.* Beaconsfield Publishers Ltd., U.K., 2000, Preface.

Taking the Case

This refers to all contact with the patient, whether in the consulting room or on the telephone. It is the process of attending to him or her, of giving your fullest attention.

The dynamics of this process involve taking, giving, receiving, allowing, following, flowing and always participating. It is more like a fluid dance than a taking down of information and I prefer to regard it as an exploration. It involves the creation of a dynamic and therapeutic relationship within which the patient is enabled to explore and meet himself and begin to move away from dis-ease.

You, the practitioner, have to be fully present. You have to listen, truly listen, and you have to observe using all of your senses. As homoeopaths we are especially interested in exploring the energy behind words, gestures and expressions.

The homoeopathic consultation provides the opportunity to explore the susceptibility of the patient. What does he attract in his life? Why? How does he react to that? How and why has he created this disease within himself?

In this exploration your own sensitivities and susceptibilities will come into play: yielding and returning create the fluid dynamic, the dance between two fields of energy.

This hopefully therapeutic encounter is a one-off event in space and time, a unique experience: don't miss it by not being fully present!

Resources
1. Brian Kaplan. *The Homeopathic Conversation; The Art of Taking the Case.* Natural Medicine Press, London, 2002.

Case Analysis

The aim of this process is to find the most homoeopathic response to the diseased patient, now. This task can be hard work, '*a very cogitative, laborious, arduous business*'. To find the unifying symptom complex amongst a morass of signs, symptoms, befallments and circumstances is not always easy, although there are equally times when nothing could be easier! The task is also potentially seductive because it can be easy to get caught up in the process, to let it become more our own process and to miss the patient!

When I think of 'case analysis' I think of onions! On the one hand is the idea of slicing through to the 'centre of the case'. On the other is the removal of 'layers' of disease, one by one, until the former healthiest state is arrived at.

Some practitioners favour one approach at the exclusion of the other: it's 'either/or'. I favour inclusivity: 'and/both'. I hope to be able to respond in the most homoeopathic way according to what is happening inside the patient, not according to my ideas of what should be happening.

So, what is the task? To find the one medicine, the simillimum, which will effect a curative response on all levels, from within outwards? Or to find a medicine, the first in a series of similars, which will effect a curing response from within each layer outwards, and in one layer of disease at a time?

It depends.

The 'simillimum' approach seems to be particularly, and often dramatically, successful when:
There is only one disease to be cured;
That one disease is an emotional one, 'spun and maintained by the soul';
That one disease has a clear aetiology or beginning.

This approach is often known as 'constitutional' or 'psychosomatic' prescribing, is underpinned by Kentian thinking and involves the creation of a 'hierarchy of symptoms'. As I understand it, this is the way of the 'classical homoeopath'.

The 'layered' approach seems to be most useful when:
There is more than one disease;
Any one of the diseases has resulted in gross pathology;
The diseases are complicated by drug treatments and suppressions;
There are a number of traumas, miasmatic attunements and circumstances to complicate matters;
The core or constitution of the person cannot be perceived because of any of the above.

This approach fits well with Hahnemannian thinking and is well demonstrated through the work of homoeopaths such as Burnett, Elmiger, Smits and Eizayaga. My hope is that a dynamic practitioner will be able to respond according to the needs of the patient.

Resources
1. Ian Watson. *A Guide to the Methodologies of Homoeopathy.* Cutting Edge Publications, Cumbria, England, 1991.

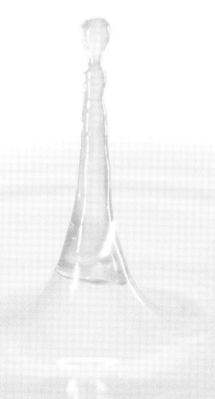

5

Part Five : The Medicines

The Law of Similars

This lies at the foundation of homoeopathic medicine. It is '*the only curative law in conformity with nature: similia similibus curentur*'. Hahnemann explains this very clearly:

'*In order to cure gently, rapidly, certainly and permanently in each case of disease, choose a medicine which can, of itself, arouse a similar suffering to the one it is supposed to cure.*' (Intro. 48)

The more there is similarity between the medicinal disease and the natural disease the greater the resonance between them, and so the greater the susceptibility of the diseased patient to the medicine and the greater the potential for cure. Another way of putting this might be that the closer the relationship between the medicine and the disease, the greater the potential for cure.

Simple.

It is clear to me that this similarity can exist at different levels within the organism and at different times. Also, according to Dr J.H. Clarke:

'It is possible to obtain the needed correspondence in a great variety of ways and degrees, and one practitioner will find it in one way and another in another.' (1)

To induce a similar disease within the life force, the medicine moves and acts in a similar way, going with the flow of the energy, not against it. In this way it cannot be suppressive.

References
1. J. H. Clarke. *A Dictionary of Practical Materia Medica.* B. Jain Publishers (P) Ltd., New Delhi, 1992, Volume 1, Preface, p. ix.

Dynamic Medicines

A dynamic disease calls for a dynamic cure, calls for a medicine which can, '*of itself, arouse a similar suffering*' in the '*spirit-like*' life force. To do this it follows that the medicine must have a '*spirit-like*' power to similarly mistune the life force, must have its own individual dynamis.

It is firstly in the provings that we begin to explore the individual dynamis of the medicine in its relationship with human beings. It is here that we begin to discover the disease-causing, and therefore disease-curing, power within each medicine.

'*...a medicine is sought which...has the power and the tendency to engender the artificial disease state most similar to that of the case of disease in question*' (Aph. 24). In terms of this power Hahnemann is clear that the medicinal disease needs to be similar and somewhat stronger than the natural one.

'*Each single case of disease is most surely, thoroughly, rapidly and permanently annihilated and lifted only by a medicine that can engender, in the human condition, a totality of symptoms that is the most complete and the most similar to the case of disease but that, at the same time, exceeds the disease in strength.*' (Aph. 27)

This '*tendency to engender*' relates to the action of the medicine, to its ability to induce similar symptoms. '*Power*' relates to quality, strength, energy, relates to the potency of the medicine. To be truly homoeopathic a medicine needs to be similar in action and in quality to the natural disease dynamis.

Hahnemann suggests that the natural disease is '*lifted*' from the awareness of the patient dynamis when this is '*seized*' or '*occupied*' by the medicinal potence. The medicinal potence '*masters the feeling of the patient*' so that the life principle can no longer experience the weaker energy of the natural disease; '*it exists no more*'. After a while the medicinal disease '*plays itself out*' and the patient returns himself to health (Aph. 29 and Aph. 45).

Again we can notice the movement of '*befallments*' and '*falling ill*' giving rise to the movement of '*lifting*'. The idea here is of falls being followed by risings, easings by dis-easings, in the undulating flow of a life.

The Simillimum

Although Hahnemann only used this word once (Aph. 56, fn.) it has come to represent the 'Holy Grail' of the homoeopath. Essentially the term means 'the best fitting' or 'most similar', 'the most homoeopathic' medicine for any case of disease. However, it has somehow come to represent the idea of the one medicine that will cure the patient of all disease and restore him to complete health by itself. It seems that, apart from an occasional acute prescription (at most), the patient will not need any other medicine for the rest of his life (other than a further dose now and again). I can only assume that this medicine will therefore reflect and cure the constitutional and miasmatic elements, the totality of all symptoms, all causations, circumstances and befallments.

This thinking is not Hahnemannian. It does not have to be Hahnemannian; I just want to be clear that it is not. Neither is it my consistent experience in practice, nor that of many successful homoeopaths.

Hahnemann writes often of people experiencing more than one disease at any one time (Aphorisms 36, 40, 43, 45). This strongly suggests the use of more than one medicine to bring about a total cure. This is especially the case when treating miasmatic diseases:

Psora '*is very seldom cured by any single anti-psoric remedy, but requires the use of several of these remedies - in the worst cases the use of quite a number of them - one after the other, for its perfect cure.*' (CD 122)

Hahnemann treated people using more than one medicine. He prescribed medicines in sequence, over time. He prescribed according to dynamic similarity and he noticed that this would change in the fluid process of cure.

Over time, many experienced practitioners have noticed patterns in prescribing, have noticed how often one medicine is followed by another in a complementing series, have noticed a relationship between certain medicines. This can be very useful in practice.

Whenever I have consciously searched for the simillimum as 'Holy Grail' I have found the search to be much more about me than the patient. As in the legend of the Grail itself, the key is in asking the question that needs to be asked and then following the process which streams from that. The outcome is the outcome, whether that is one medicine or a series of medicines.

One Medicine

'The true medical art practitioner already finds in quite simple medicines, employed singly and un-mixed, all that he could wish for: artificial disease potences which are able to completely over-tune natural diseases by homoeopathic power, to extinguish them for the feeling of the life principle and to permanently cure them. Therefore, it will never occur to the true medical art practitioner to administer more than one simple medicinal substance at one time as a remedy, in accordance with the wise saying that it is wrong to use complex means when simple ones will suffice.' (Aph. 274)

One medicine at a time is good science. It means that we have the possibility of finding out what it will do within that one individual. This is crucial information in the process of health restoration.

One medicine at one time is not the same as one medicine for all time. One medicine at one time does not exclude another medicine at another time.

A simple, single medicine has been fully proven as such, whereas a combination has not. We cannot know how this will impinge upon the life force.

Keep it simple.

Dynamizing the Medicines

'*The homoeopathic medical art develops…the internal, spirit-like medicinal powers of crude substances*' (Aph. 269) through a multi-step process involving dilution and succussion or trituration. This dynamic power to alter the state of health, to mistune the life force, is latent and, before Hahnemann, was unnoticeable in many substances. This life power is 'sleeping' in rock, such as Silica; 'dreaming' in plant, such as Pulsatilla; 'awakening' in animal, such as Lachesis; and 'becoming conscious of itself' in man, such as Lac humanum.

A dynamized medicine has a purely dynamic effect, rather than a molecular one. The dynamized medicine exerts its influence upon the force that moves the molecules. '*The dynamic powers of these substances mainly have an influence on the life principle.*' (Aph. 269) My understanding is that the dynamis takes up the medicinal influence and instinctively organises the most appropriate response.

Homoeopathic medicines are not '*mere dilutions*'. Through the processes of trituration and succussion, material substances are somehow de-materialised, energised, potentised, '*spiritized.*' (Aph. 269, fn. b)

'*Homoeopathic dynamizations are processes by which the medicinal properties, which are latent in natural substances while in their crude state, become aroused, and then become enabled to act in an almost spiritual manner on our life.*' (CD xxiii)

This is especially the case during trituration, each step of which involves grinding the medicinal substance and lactose with a pestle and mortar for one hour. Try it yourself. Find out what energy is involved!

Action of the Medicines

I understand that the medicine is taken up by the life force in the same way as disease potences, '*in one single moment*'. As we have seen:

'*Each life-impinging potence, each medicine, alters the tuning of the life force more or less and arouses a certain alteration of a person's condition for a longer or a shorter time. This is termed the* **initial action**. *While the initial action is a product of both the medicinal energy and the life force, it* **belongs more** *to the impinging potence (of the medicine). Our life force strives to oppose this impinging action with its own energy. This back-action belongs to our sustentive power of life and is an automatic function of it, called the* '**after-action** *or* **counter-action**.' (Aph. 63)

The generative aspect of the life force allows the medicinal potence, '*impinging from without*', to make an impression upon it. Because the medicinal disease is similar but '*somewhat stronger*' than the original natural disease, the life force may be slightly '*overtuned*' and the patient may experience a degree of homoeopathic aggravation. '*This aggravation is so similar to the original disease that it appears to the patient to be an aggravation of his own malady. In fact, it is nothing other than a highly similar medicinal disease that is somewhat stronger than the original malady.*' (Aph. 157)

The sustentive aspect of the life force is then stimulated to oppose the medicinal potence with its own energy and return the patient towards health. This is the 're-bound' which we look for in response to the curative medicine. In good homoeopathic treatment the degree of '*counter-action*' is generally just sufficient '*to again raise the condition up to the natural healthy state*' (Aph. 112). This is the law of the minimum dose: the amount or degree of medicinal stimulation necessary to induce a curative response is always the least. This involves a consideration of both potency and dose.

The fluid mechanism described above relates to the processes of cure, disease and proving. It is not always possible to be sure which symptoms are due to the initial action or to the counter-action.

Provings

This is the process through which we enter into relationship with our medicines. A medicinal potence impinges upon human life and we explore what happens as a result. A proving is the country of '*pure experience*' and, if you enjoy good health, I would encourage you to participate in such an exploration at least once.

Each medicine is unique.

'*Every medicine exhibits particular actions in the human body which do not come about in exactly the same way from any other medicinal substance of a different kind.*' (Aph. 118) '*Therefore the medicines upon which the life and death, the disease and health of human beings depend must be exactly, painstakingly distinguished from one another.*' (Aph. 120)

Anyone who has been involved in the collation of information gathered in a proving will fully understand the word '*painstaking*'! Symptoms induced in a proving are almost entirely due to the primary (initial) action of the medicinal potence upon the life force. This is the same in the process of disease. The secondary (after) action is '*seldom or almost never in the least to be sensed*' (Aph. 112).

In a proving we are exploring what kind of dynamic mistunement, what kind of medicinal disease, will be induced in healthy humans. This is the way to compile a '*true materia medica*' (Aph. 143). It is also a way of finding out about ourselves, both as individuals and as parts of the collective. Within human beings are many places, in heart, mind and body, that only come into awareness through suffering. These places can become known during a proving.

Hahnemann tells us that taking part in a proving is good for our health: '*The prover's organism becomes more seasoned (hardened) against everything that is detrimental. His health becomes more invariable; he becomes more robust, as all experience teaches.*' (Aph. 141, fn.) He certainly set us a good example by dying at the age of 85 with all his faculties intact, married to a younger woman and healthier and happier than he had ever been!

My own experience is that a proving is like entering in to the gymnasium of the dynamis: I know I am in for a work-out, and maybe a little pain, but I will be stronger for it.

Resources
1. Jeremy Sherr. *The Dynamics and Methodology of Homoeopathic Provings.* Dynamis Books, 1994.

Hering's Observations on Cure

1. 'Pain is relieved from above downwards.'
2. 'Diseases improve from within outwards.'
3. 'Symptoms disappear in the same order as they appeared, the most important or vital organs being relieved first, then the less important ones, and finally the mucous membranes and the skin.' (1)

Point three refers to a 'determined disease', a simple example of which would be an acute infectious disease. It makes sense that this would also apply to ideogenic diseases.

The common observation, first made by Kent, that 'symptoms disappear in the reverse order of their coming' applies mainly in the treatment of chronic miasmatic diseases, or of successive and suppressed diseases suffered by the patient throughout his life. In these cases it is also observed that symptoms re-appear in the reverse order of their appearance in the process of re-winding back to the healthiest state.

Other writers have since added the observation that, in the process of cure, the disease focus moves from more important organs to less important ones. Also, it often seems that these changes in disease focus move from more dynamic organs (such as the liver) to less dynamic ones (such as the gall bladder).

'Even the most superficial observer will not fail in recognising this law of order.' (1)

References
1. Constantine Hering, writing in the prologue to Hahnemann's *The Chronic Diseases,* New York, 1845; as discussed in *Treatise on Homoeopathic Medicine*: Francisco Xavier Eizayaga, Ediciones Marcel, Buenos Aires, 1991, p. 102.

The Law of Cure

From a single-celled beginning in my mother's womb, through the foetal uncurling in her belly to my torrential birth head downwards, I have lived upon this Earth. I have grown up and crashed down, gone down further into myself, found a bottom line and began again to grow, more in the direction of maturity (hopefully!) I will die, and I can only hope to fulfil my potential, to realise the full potency of my being.

This unfolding of myself, this stretching out to my limit, echoes the movement of the universe outwards from centre. 'Like a current of energy that discharges itself from the centre, our life cycle ends with the dispersion of the elements that make up our physical body.' (1)

This electrical charge arises in the quantum field, is sourced by the field, is organised into my life by the dynamis, and returns to the field when I die. 'This progression from centre to periphery, that is, from embodiment in a living unit towards dispersion or death, is what we call the law of cure.' (1)

'The purpose of the law of cure is not to prevent death, but to allow death to come smoothly and normally, thus allowing the individual to fulfil the highest purpose of existence - to become aware of his metaphysical relationship with the whole of existence.' (1)

The ripples disperse on the surface of the lake, the river returns to the sea, the coalescence returns to the field. A life expands to its limit and then contracts to its end. Energy is expressed, dissipated and returned to the one source. Suppressions, repressions and oppressions may dam, block or hinder this natural flow of energy during a life. This is disease. Homoeopathic medicines gently allow the individual flow to continue. When the energy of a life is flowing easily no medicine is needed.

I love the passion and beauty in Paschero's writing and I have included him here because he inspires me and enhances my understanding. However, the Law of Cure is clearly stated: *'similia similibus curentur (let similars be cured by similars')*. This is *'the only curative law in conformity with nature'* (Intro. 48).

Perhaps the observations of Hering and Paschero relate more to direction within the curative process than to the law which governs it.

References
1. T. P. Paschero. *Homoeopathy.* Beaconsfield Publishers Ltd., U.K., 2000, Ch. 3.

Does it Work?

Yes.
It does.

As long as there is sufficient similarity between the disease state and the medicinal state, then homoeopathic medicines will induce a response in a curative direction.

There is a mass of anecdotal evidence from millions of people who are not stupid or easily fooled. There are now over two hundred well-verified clinical trials, and at least five meta-analyses of such trials, which demonstrate the effectiveness of homoeopathy (1). There is enough evidence. This question has been answered.

And it is generally safe!

How does it work?
As yet, we don't know.
And: mainstream medical science does not yet have a context or model within which to find out how it works.
And: we were prescribing opium and its derivatives for several hundred years before we knew how it worked.
And: we still don't know what happens to people when we anaesthetize them.
And: work in many different fields, by such scientists as Benveniste (2), Milgrom (3) and Emoto (4) is moving us closer to an answer to how homoeopathy works.

Meanwhile mainstream medicine is not as safe and effective as we thought it would be. If it were, we'd all be practising it!

Patience!

References

1. David Reilly. *Homeopathy: Increasing Scientific Validation.* Alternative Therapies, March/April 2005, Vol. 11, No. 2.
2. Lynne McTaggart. *The Field - The Quest for the Secret Force of the Universe.* HarperCollins Publishers Ltd., 2001, p. 60-73.
3. Lionel Milgrom. *Reconciling Science with Homeopathy: Towards a Calculus of Cure?* The Homeopath, No. 93, Spring 2004, pp. 8-12.
4. Masaru Emoto. *Messages From Water.* I.H.M. General Research Institute, Hado Kyoikusha Co. Ltd., 2002.

Resources

1. Society of Homeopaths Website. *Key Clinical Trials in Homeopathy.* www.homeopathy-soh.org

Placebo

This is an 'inactive' drug or 'sham' treatment given to placate or please the patient. The patient trusts the practitioner and believes that an active and genuine drug or treatment has been given, and reacts as if this were so. Orthodox medical thinking suggests that this belief may induce a psychosomatic benefit within the patient. How this happens is not understood. In the Randomised Clinical Trial, the gold standard of clinical research, placebo is supposed to represent the known. It is the blank against which treatments are tested. Actually it is still a mystery.

Any medical practitioner, of any kind, who does not acknowledge the potential beneficial power of placebo is a fool. It has been observed for centuries.

To suggest that homoeopathic medicine works purely because of this placebo effect is also foolish. A scenario commonly encountered in homoeopathic medical practice makes my point:

A man develops a health problem. Sooner or later he takes this problem to his doctor, his G.P., for diagnosis and treatment. Like most people in twenty-first century western culture, he has an inherent belief that this is the best, indeed only, course of action. He has started out with the belief that 'scientific medicine' will cure him. He has no reason to doubt this.

After several diagnoses, several visits to 'the consultant', and after maybe half a dozen prescriptions of 'state of the art drugs' (some of which cause 'side effects') he is no better. He begins to feel disillusioned. He says things like 'I can't believe that in this day and age they can't find out what's wrong and sort me out!' His belief in 'scientific medicine' has been gradually undermined, usually over quite some time. In desperation he visits a homoeopath and, after an hour or so of conversation, is given a single plain white tablet. The measure of his belief in the treatment is expressed through his exclamation of 'Is that it?'

Reluctantly, yet still desperate for relief, he decides to 'give it a go.' On his follow-up visit he declares that nothing has changed: 'I am no better.' After another conversation the homoeopath agrees that nothing has changed, yet - on the basis of some further information elucidated from the patient - would like to prescribe a different plain white tablet. The patient decides to 'give it one last shot'.

Two weeks later he calls to say 'I don't know what you gave me this time but my symptoms got a little worse for a few days and have now all gone. I can't believe it!'

His improvement is apparently due to the placebo effect! Doesn't make a great deal of sense does it?

It seems to me that the G.P. had the best chance to make use of the placebo effect, the consultant the next best chance and the homoeopath the least.

And babies and unconscious people apparently benefit from placebo. Oh, and animals.

Water

When I think about life force I often think about water too. Water is an elegant and eloquent metaphor for energy. Water flows. Water is the most definitively flowing phenomenon in our world. It flows from the mountains, down rivers, to the sea. It floats across our skies as cloud, it pours as rain and it swirls as snow. Water streams through rainforest, spills from our eyes and floods the land as tsunami. Life force also flows: as skein, swarm and shoal; as volcano, savannah and blood-steam; as galaxy and crowd. Human life can seemingly evaporate in battle or disaster as easily as frost off a sun-warmed rock. And, like life force, it's the very fluidity of water that seems to give it strength:

> 'In heavy snow
> The pine branch breaks,
> While the willow
> Simply bends.' (1)

Water is fundamental to Life; it is the medium through which Life expresses itself most easily and luxuriantly. All life processes take place in, through, or because of, water. Yet water seems to be such a simple thing, and has all its virtues simply by being itself! Water nourishes and destroys, separates and brings together. It flows from the highest to the lowest, filling up and moving on, always finding its way through, under, over or around. Always taking the path of least resistance, always seeking its own level.

Water creates its own cycle of movement from the high cloud to the rain, through the streams and rivers to the ocean and, via the invisible evaporation process, back to cloud.

Water also expresses itself through differing densities, through solid, liquid and vapour. Its patterns of flow are in everything; ripples, bubbles, cascades, swirls, eddies, waves and tides. These can be observed in blood flow and crystal, growth rings and bone, in population explosions, in driftwood, in the lines on an old man's face.

Around 70% of the surface of the Earth is water. A human being is 70 - 80% water. As citizens we are each individual cells in the greater organism of life force so fluidly organized as the Blue Planet. As much as there is commonality to human being, so there is individuality; just as every wave separates out from the ocean in its individual rush to the shore, so every snowflake is unique.

And snowflakes have been photographed, their beautiful crystal structures revealed. And then they have been melted and re-frozen, and photographed again. And each time the snowflake has resumed its original, individual shape. Clearly there is an organizing principle or dynamis here, some light or energy, something '*spirit-like*' in the water.

Water.

Maybe this is why I think that the research of people like Benveniste, Milgrom and Emoto (2) will eventually reveal how our medicines influence so profoundly.

References
1. Taoist poem.
2. See 'Does It Work?'

Story

A girl child was born in 1950.
There was cancer in her family history.

At the age of six months she yielded to the dynamic influence associated with a microorganism known as *Bordetella pertussis*, and she developed respiratory symptoms, most notable of which was a pronounced whooping cough. After some time she returned to health.

As a little girl she was often described as being bubbly, sensitive and caring.

At the age of twelve her father, whom she had experienced as a tyrant who constantly criticised and undermined her, died and left her alone. She yielded to the very powerful dynamic influence of this event and an impression was made upon her; she felt deep loss, pain, grief and rage. She cried for an hour or so on hearing the news and then 'had to be strong' for her mother. Her reaction was to close down emotionally, to brood inwardly. She did not return to her healthiest state.

Over the next thirty years or so she lived her life. The most common theme throughout this time was that she entered into relationships with a number of different men, all of whom undermined her in different ways, all of whom then left her, alone. And each time she was left, alone, she felt something deeply and reacted by closing off her heart more and more and more because she 'had to look after' her three children. Which she did.

In her mid-forties she was suddenly diagnosed as having a tumour, 'like a small egg', in her right breast. She yielded to the dynamic influence of this brutal diagnosis and an impression was made upon her; she felt something, deeply. She was later to describe that feeling as 'a shattering'. Her reaction was to seek holistic health care, and so she arrived in your consulting room.

And you took the case, you received the case, you explored the case. You yielded to the dynamic of this woman, her story, her pathology, and she made an impression upon you. You felt something, and you noticed something, and you thought something, and you returned with a dynamic prescription: Conium, and she went away.

And she yielded to the dynamic influence of this similar medicine and, over some time, she returned to say that the breast lump had disappeared and that she was feeling great relief.

And you explored some more together and you yielded to a slightly different dynamic, and she made a different impression upon you. And you felt something, and you noticed something, and you thought something, and you returned with a simple question:
'Are you happy?'
And tears welled up in her eyes and she said, 'No'.
And you asked her, very gently, 'Why not?'
And she smiled a little smile as tears trickled down her cheeks and she whispered, 'I don't know'.
And you prescribed Carcinosin, and she went away.

And she yielded to the dynamic influence of the medicine and, after some time, she returned with brighter spirits, a more positive attitude and a new boyfriend. In time, this man began to undermine her: in time she told him to 'Go away'. And this happened several times, and then she came to see you and presented an aspect of herself that you had not experienced before. She was withdrawn, resentful, bitterly expressing how unfair life was and how, despite all her hard work on herself, all she seemed to attract were men who ended up abusing her in some way. And she hated them.

And you yielded to her dynamic and she made a different impression upon you, and you felt something, and you noticed something, and you thought something and you returned with a different dynamic prescription: Natrum muriaticum, and she went away.

And she yielded to the dynamic influence of this medicine and, over some time, she returned with symptoms that she had experienced before. She returned with tears and an anger that she expressed. In time, she returned with a new man friend, a man who was treating her with respect and with love. And she shone!

And she told you how she was feeling more like her real self, an old self that somehow felt new. And she felt both excited and afraid. And you were able to explain to her, in a way that made sense to her, how she was no longer susceptible to a certain kind of man: how she had first of all changed her reaction to such men, and had then stopped attracting them into her life. A vacuum had been filled, a wound had been healed, a loss had been honoured and integrated and she had returned herself to her healthiest state. And you applauded her!

And as she left, she kissed you on the cheek in thanks. And you yielded to the dynamic of that kiss, and an impression was made upon you. And you felt something, and you noticed something, and you thought something. And you went to see your next patient.

You returned to your work touched by its simplicity, by its power, and its depth.

End

Medicine flows
And ebbs and flows
And medicines flow
Singly
Or in beautiful sequences
From one to the other
In the process of cure.

Allow

Follow

Flow on

With confidence.

Keep it simple.

Notes